Praise for *

'Henika is a wise, embodied sou
on the ancient wisdom of Ta
makes it accessible and inviting

'Henika's work is liberating and authentic. She is a visionary, channeling wisdom from our Indian culture making it relevant for these times. She doesn't shy away from dealing with challenging and sometimes taboo topics like shame, trauma, fear, and stress. In fact, she turns toward these challenging experiences and invites us into a gateway to transformation with her work and words. With her stories, practices, and wisdom, she gives us inspiring and useful tools. *Sensual* will make a powerful addition to your bookshelf, unlocking experiences and emotions to live your practice.'

'I heartily recommend Henika's wise and friendly guide to tantra. This book is exactly what's needed right now. Henika's authentic insights and personal connection to these precious teachings make them super accessible for everyone. Every human with senses to feel the world needs this book!'

'Henika's book is a beautiful journey into rediscovering depth and connection in all areas of your life. Her words and practices will help you to find your spark and feel alive again.'

SENSUAL

SENSUAL

Connect Deeply, Express Freely, Love Intimately

HENIKA PATEL

HAY HOUSE

Carlsbad, California • New York City
London • Sydney • New Delhi

Published in the United Kingdom by:
Hay House UK Ltd, The Sixth Floor, Watson House
54 Baker Street, London W1U 7BU
Tel: +44 (0)20 3927 7290; www.hayhouse.co.uk

Published in the United States of America by:
Hay House LLC, PO Box 5100, Carlsbad, CA 92018-5100
Tel: (1) 760 431 7695 or (800) 654 5126; www.hayhouse.com

Published in Australia by:
Hay House Australia Ltd, 18/36 Ralph St, Alexandria NSW 2015
Tel: (61) 2 9669 4299; www.hayhouse.com.au

Published in India by:
Hay House Publishers India, Muskaan Complex,
Plot No.3, B-2, Vasant Kunj, New Delhi 110 070
Tel: (91) 11 4176 1620; www.hayhouse.co.in

Text © Henika Patel, 2024

The moral rights of the author have been asserted.

The information given in this book should not be treated as a substitute for professional medical advice; always consult a medical practitioner. Any use of information in this book is at the reader's discretion and risk. Neither the author nor the publisher can be held responsible for any loss, claim or damage arising out of the use, or misuse, of the suggestions made, the failure to take medical advice or for any material on third-party websites.

A catalogue record for this book is available from the British Library.

Tradepaper ISBN: 978-1-4019-7583-8
E-book ISBN: 978-1-83782-052-8
Audiobook ISBN: 978-1-83782-053-5

Interior Illustrations: 1, 99, 185: Shutterstock; 42, 75, 77, 136, 245: Jade Ho; 78, 80, 83, 85, 87, 90, 92: Shutterstock/OkPic; 160: Shutterstock/Trikona

10 9 8 7 6 5 4 3 2 1

Printed in the United States of America

This product uses responsibly sourced papers and/or recycled materials. For more information, see www.hayhouse.com.

To my sweet sister Jalpa,
whose loss taught me how to live.

Vigyan Bhairav Tantra – Yukti 32

Every perception is an invitation into revelation.
Hearing, seeing, smelling, tasting, touching –
Ways of knowing creation,
Transmissions of electric realization,
The deepest reality is always right here.

Encircled by splendor, in the center of the sphere
Meditate where the body thrills
To currents of intimate communion
Follow your senses to the end and beyond
Into the heart of space.

THE RADIANCE SUTRAS, LORIN ROCHE[1]

Contents

Introduction

Do you remember the last time you felt a spark for life? Eyes bright and curious while the moon moved across the sky, curious as to how the night might unravel. Jumping in puddles and getting dirty. Slow days, watching raindrops chase one another across the window. Fast days, rolling down a hill in summer. Grass stains down your jeans and sand in your hair. Crying when it hurt and longing for playtime. The twinge in your body as someone you found attractive passed by. Flutters in your belly as you daydreamed about the moment you'd see them again. Savoring the scent of a lover on your skin. The meal that you never wanted to end. Sticking your hand out the car window to feel the breeze brush through your fingers. And finally, laying your head down to rest in a warm bed, eager for it to begin all over again. Moments where even the mundane is filled with a magic, the heart fills with a zest for life, and the mind computes its infinite possibilities.

One day, I woke up and I didn't feel it anymore. That spark was gone, and I didn't know where to find it again. This one day turned into two months, and two months turned into years. Curious days transformed into a cycle of 'work, eat, sleep, repeat.'

The monotony of life had become so normal that I didn't even realize I had set my days on autopilot, driving my life like those trips in the car you look back at and barely remember. If those days had a color, they would have been beige, with little left to distinguish one from another. I looked around the morning commute – a flurry of white, black, and grey overcoats – and sat wondering if the other people I was crammed into the carriage with felt it, too: a disconnect with myself, my work, and my relationships, coupled with an unsatisfied desire to feel deeply alive within it all again.

Lacking the vocabulary to express any of this, I found a way to numb my pain and emptiness. My quest toward rediscovering that spark hadn't yet begun. On the surface, I appeared to be a highly social, successful, optimistically positive extrovert. I had studied English and French law, and I was living abroad. Despite my busy schedule, I was the friend who always said yes to going out. Call me Monday, Tuesday, Thursday, Sunday, any day – it didn't matter! I had short but thrilling relationships – holiday romances filled with hot sun, sand, and romance. They lasted long enough to give me that warm, fuzzy feeling inside and short enough so that I never had to get too vulnerable. I'd created my own perfect concoction of getting naked on the outside but staying fully dressed on the inside.

I also started taking the frustrations of my everyday life out on my body and wallet. I escaped into the world of intoxicants in the hope of finding freedom and connection. I bought material things that filled my house but didn't fill my heart. I changed countries, jobs, and locations to distract myself from facing the truth that was bubbling away inside – that I was full of grief and unprocessed experiences. I was seeking the 'shiny new' feeling of excitement so much that I couldn't stay still – in one place or situation or relationship – long enough to feel my emotions or experience the depths of connection that only came with the sweet surrender into time. And in the midst of conjuring up these avoidance tactics, I lost touch with the last strand of myself, my spirit.

An incredible facade and character called Henika had emerged, speaking the lines that her society, her family, her culture, her education, and her peers had written for her, because she couldn't find the words to write her own script. As each day passed, the voices of others grew louder, and I knew myself less and less. A friend asked me, 'What ice cream do you like?' A colleague asked me, 'What's your favorite film?' A fellow party-goer asked me, 'So, what do you like in bed?' I was completely thrown by the first two questions and deeply ashamed to respond to the last one. Stumbling over my words, I was glad the bartender arrived in time to distract me with another round of drinks.

Bit by bit, a deep depression sank its teeth into me. This wasn't the life I'd imagined. I was left wondering how I got here – and more importantly: How was I going to get out?

Sensual Numbness

One cold afternoon, my then-partner and I were attempting to 'make love,' when I realized I could not feel it anymore. My pelvis, my heart, my mind – *everything* felt numb. It made me question: If love was to be 'made,' what were the ingredients and why was my recipe not working? I'd studied and achieved the relative health, wealth, and status that society had proclaimed would set me on the path to fulfillment and happiness. I found my partner attractive, kind, gentle, sweet, and caring. We did everything together – I thought that was love. So, why was my cake so stale? I stayed just a little bit longer in that relationship to experience the immediate attraction fade into a game of attachments and comfort.

As confusing as it was, I look back with deep respect for that relationship because it became the catalyst that showed me I was stuck in a rut of patterns so deep, it was going to hurt to rip myself out. I was left with the same questions that had been nagging me for months: Where did I go? Where did she go? She was the one who effortlessly flirted with life; she was the one who was capable of feeling and nurturing the spark I had lost. It was this absence of love and aliveness, as well as my sense that I could reclaim both, that plunged me into my journey with sensuality.

And it all started with this simple question: Why is my pelvis numb?

It wasn't an easy question to answer. Naively, I believed it was just about the sex, and that a simple fix to my intimate relations would be the cure. Maybe a new toy? New lingerie? New haircut? An exciting fling? A quick trip to a different country? But somehow, I understood that no amount of 'new' things or distractions would be a big enough Band-Aid. When a series of Google searches couldn't give me the answers I was looking for, I set off on my own course to discover how to turn my mind, body, and spirit back online.

I remember being at lunch with some girlfriends and asking if anyone had experienced empty sex or numbness in their pelvis. I was left with an even emptier stare. The quick dive out of the conversation left me feeling alone and unsatisfied. Back then, when a girl in her early twenties began to ask those around her about 'unfulfilling sex and numb vaginas,' she'd get stuck in the fear that she might be considered a slut on one hand or frigid on the other. Maybe she should just get some lube, buy a vibrator, and have a good shag to put an end to it all. At the time, I didn't consider that perhaps my friends' discomfort in talking about sex and their bodies reflected a wider repression in society, or that the numbness could have been an indication of something deeper going on. When neither search engine nor friends could answer the questions I had, it marked the beginnings of a research or (me-search) so consuming that it would eventually become my life's work, first to turn my own body back online — and then to realize there must also be other people out there, searching for their spark, whom I could share the answers with.

Over time, I realized that my numb pelvis mirrored a numbness in my feelings, my work, my relationships, and just about every other category of my life. I came to a jarring conclusion: What I experienced in the bedroom was a direct reflection of my life outside of it. I craved tasting, seeing, smelling, feeling, hearing, as well as touching life with depth and connection. I wanted meals that made my mouth water, kisses with no expectations, the experience of getting lost in the music and walking with no destination in mind. I hungered for spontaneity and the beauty I knew was possible within life. I wanted to feel alive. The quest for finding my spark had begun, and it was about far more than sex — it was about learning how to live embodied in the reality of the world, rather than escaping from it. I was searching for how to live sensually.

What Is Sensuality?

Language gives context to the way we experience the world. Metaphorically, it is the frame in which the picture of our life hangs. Comprehensive definitions of the word *sensual* are hard to come by, and they usually point to the same awkward reactions I received from my girlfriends when I began to talk about my numbness. The dictionary definition of *sensual* is 'relating to or involving a gratification of the senses and physical, especially sexual, pleasure.' The definition does well in speaking to the senses before making the unfortunate mistake of lumping sensuality together with gratification, pleasure, and sex.

I've spent a lot of time on sensuality – enough to untangle it and earn several advanced qualifications in the subject! And my message is this: Sensuality is not the same as sex.

Although sex almost always involves sensuality, sensuality doesn't always have to involve sex. Sensuality is not just about pleasure and self-gratification; it is about feeling all of our emotions more deeply so that we can connect and express more freely. It is not just about our genitals; it is about knowing our body, mind, and spirit more intimately through our sensations. It is less about *per*forming for others and more about *in*forming ourselves about how our sensations reveal moment to moment who we are, offer us a guide to our intuitive wisdom, and indicate to us what we need to live a fulfilled life. Where most definitions of sensuality fail to value it as a powerful key to self-knowledge, joy, and well-being, it has lost its place in the muddied waters where shame, sex, and society are all swimming.

Still, our languages and history are rich with definitions of sensuality. Late Latin used the term *sensualitatem*, which was regarded as 'the capacity for sensation.' In Latin, *sensualis* meant 'endowed with feeling.' In mid-14th century France, sensuality was considered the part of a human life that is associated with the senses and gave rise to the modern verb *sentir*, meaning 'to feel.' Halfway across the world, in India and the Vedic and Tantric traditions, sensual energy was regarded as *shakti*, which translates to 'dynamic creative power,' and could be cultivated for and within oneself as a tool for healing, spiritual growth, and creativity. (Tellingly, Shakti is also a name for the dynamic creative power of the universe which brings it into manifest form.)

As we moved into the 17th century, with the rise of colonization spreading religious values from the West into indigenous communities, sensuality was conflated with animal instincts, sin, savagery, sex, and selfish gratification, rather than a spiritual path in which our sensations and sensual energy connected us to source and spirit, known as Shakti. Since then, sensuality has largely been repressed, commodified to sell goods, and robbed of its true potency in our world today.

In our contemporary lives, many of us may have internalized that our sensual nature is in some way sinful, that it is 'too much' and 'too dangerous,' or 'too scary' to embody, or that it could expose and endanger us. Many people who explored their sensuality in their younger years at some point or other end up retiring it or backburnering it behind other priorities, such as career and family, etc. Some of us consider sensual living to be an unnecessary indulgence whose pursuit is selfish hedonism. Others of us may have never felt that sensual spark or even believed we are worthy of feeling it. We might fear that if we engage in sensual expression, we'll be labeled as provocative, our choices will be judged, and our actions will be hypersexualized. We might have only ever worn sensuality as a piece of underwear for others and never experienced how it can serve as a source of self-nourishment and spiritual evolution for ourselves.

I myself have tugged and torn and grappled with all of these feelings, and what I've come to learn is that sensuality is the pathway to a life of deep fulfillment; it is the spark we get to experience in embodied form, when we live fully through the senses. It allows us to root into the world, rather than trying to escape from it – to be in this world and of it, through our skin and our stretch marks, through our awe and our anger, through all the things that make us human. Our five senses are gateways to knowing ourselves, others, and the world around us with the deepest intimacy. They help us to see the sacred in each sunset, and allow our interactions and experiences with the material world to become a prayer.

Thus, the intention of this book is to shift gears from living in our minds to experiencing the world through our senses, so that we can open ourselves to love more deeply, express more freely, and connect to all of life more intimately.

So, How Did I Get Here?

As a first-generation Indian woman growing up in Britain, with an artist turned monk for a father and a mother whose family migrated from Uganda, I have spent much of my life translating between countries and continents by being immersed in the spiritual traditions and cultural concepts that have flourished through these migrations.

Between the Eastern philosophy and spiritual practices I found in my home to the understanding of the demands of growing up, being educated, and living in the Western world, I hope to offer you, the reader, a bridge between both worlds. While searching for my spark, and studying the practices, philosophies, psychology, and tools to turn my body back online, I found something much vaster – my sensuality and my spirit.

I started writing a blog about the results I was getting and realized that there are others out there who are searching for the same. That's when the School of Sensual Arts (SOSA) was born. I created it as an institution to connect soul and spirit with sensual living and share all the practices I have learned along the way. SOSA now serves thousands of individuals and couples from around the world every year, through our online community, courses, and in-person retreats.

Because I'm a human who identifies as a female she/her, the lens of my personal stories and experiences will be shaped by my lived experience. Please know that whoever you are, whatever body you are in, whatever color your skin, you are welcome here and this information is for you. Sensuality both encompasses and transcends categories of race, gender, class, sexual orientation, and other markers of identity, because it belongs to us all. With this in mind, I write these words to the best of my understanding, as an offering from my heart, to share this knowledge with even a single soul whom I can help to feel less alone in their journey of reclaiming aliveness through sensuality, a topic that has remained in the shadows for too long. Indeed, these are the very words I wish I'd had in my darkest days of feeling numb and disconnected.

In this book, I hope to clear misconceptions about sensual living by sharing what I learned from traveling the world to train with esteemed and expert teachers and guides, as well as through my own ancestral and cultural practices. Many of the practices and philosophies I share have been cultivated in India, China, and other parts of Asia, yet they belong to all of us — because to feel and to sense is our natural birthright as humans. And although this book and its practices are largely influenced by my study of Tantra and familial lineage of Sanatana Dharma (the precolonial name for Hinduism), I do not espouse one particular school of thought, religion, or doctrine. Instead, I have chosen to weave together all that I have studied to overcome obstacles and reignite our sensuality across the subjects of spirituality, embodiment, and psychology.

With a drive to help move Tantra from a widely misunderstood and culturally appropriated subject, I'll share with you its origins, ancient texts, and mythology. You'll meet the Tantric gods and goddesses who underpin the core values and philosophies of Tantra through the ancient art of storytelling. In this way, my hope is that, in addition to sharing my own personal and professional journey with clients, as well as some very practical exercises, I'll introduce you to the roots and principles behind them.

How to Use This Book

We're about to get started on the road to expansion, so if you're ready, strap in and read this book with your whole body. Notice the sensations as your eyes cross the page. Feel into what resonates, what doesn't, and how your body responds to each sentence. Interact with these pages, highlight them when you see anything of interest, write down questions when you're curious to learn more, and speak back to me as I share these words with you. Explore what resonates, what's new, and what interests you.

The book is divided into three parts: The first will help you discover your natural sensuality; the second helps to combat the four most common blocks to deepening into your sensuality; and the third shares four ways to use your sensuality to empower your life, in the bedroom and beyond!

To bring you back into the sensual home of your body, I invite you to make use of not only the principles and stories of sensuality that I offer, but also the many practices in this book that have impacted the lives of the thousands of people who have passed through the School of Sensual Arts (SOSA). For if you read this book without taking part in any of the practices, sensuality will remain a concept in your mind rather than an experience in your body and life.

Therefore, the best way to get the most out of this book is not just to read the information, but to embody it — for through these pages, you will discover sounds you've never heard, smells you've never smelled, sights you've never seen, textures you've never touched, flavors you've never tasted, and a connection to your sensual self you never previously imagined.

So, even if the practices feel new, silly, or strange, be open to the invitations, as this is a book that's as much for the body as it is for the mind. Take pride in picking up this book and holding it in your hands, sensual one — knowing that as you flip through each page, you take one further step toward accessing your sensual wisdom.

To join the SOSA online community and access lots of great resources to help you on your sensual journey, please visit:

www.schoolofsensualarts.co.uk

A world of potential awaits you. Welcome to your sensual revolution.

Henika

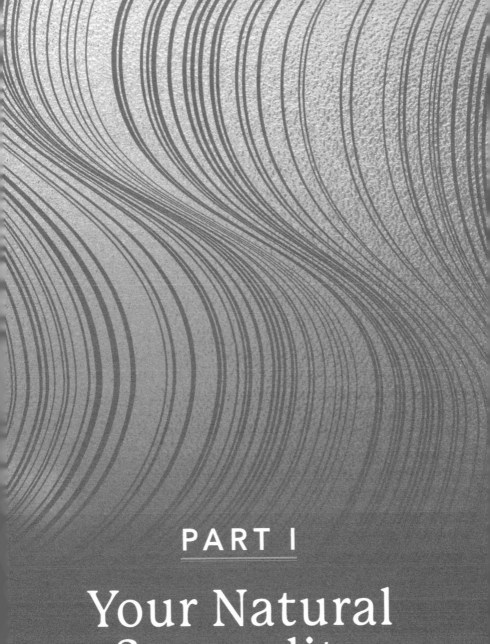

PART I

Your Natural Sensuality

Are we born a sensual being or do we become one? In this part, we'll be exploring this question together.

The premise I introduce, which is vital throughout this entire book, is that sensuality is a natural superpower you were born with. We'll look at the five instruments to sensual connection, as well as the development of sensuality over the course of your life. We'll also examine our innate sensual power through the widely misunderstood lens of Tantra, busting myths and tracing the origins of ancient practices.

We'll explore why our sensuality changes throughout the month by exploring its cyclical nature, which will lead us more intimately to the experiences our body might be desiring on a daily basis. Finally, we'll set off to explore the Sensual Rivermap that will be the framework for the SENSFUL Method and further practices that will empower our sensuality throughout Parts II and III of the book.

For now, we'll take this first step forward on our journey to understand our unapologetic, fully expressed sensual spirit.

CHAPTER 1

Knowing Your Sensuality

The Chinese Taoist philosopher Laozi once said, 'Watch your thoughts, they become your words; watch your words, they become your actions; watch your actions, they become your habits; watch your habits, they become your character; watch your character, it becomes your destiny.'

So, let's take one step back: What makes up a thought? It is our perception. And what makes up our perception? It is the information delivered from our sense organs. If our thoughts become our destiny, then our senses unravel extraordinary gateways to understanding all of life, which rests beneath our thoughts, beyond our words. Our senses introduce us to a new and potentially unexplored landscape of potential in which we can know ourselves with the deepest intimacy.

In this chapter, we will explore the Tantric approach to the senses, why our sensual development is so important, and how it can provide us with a vehicle for navigating the terrain of our own physical, emotional, and spiritual evolution.

Starting here, I propose that we move from being 'mind-ful,' or watching the thoughts through meditation, to being 'sense-ful,' or watching the senses through sensation.

Waking Up with the Senses

I am a daughter of Bhadran, which sits in the west of India, in a state called Gujarat. Our town's *Kul-devi* or 'patron saint' is Bhadrakali, a compassionate form of the eminent Tantric figurehead, Goddess Kali.

My father was born there and lived down a small cul-de-sac street, growing up with many of the people I now call aunties and uncles. My grandfather worked for the local government, and my grandmother was raising six children. She was known for swimming laps of the local lake in her *sari*. In his morning break, my grandfather would pick freshly scented jasmine flowers from the manicured gardens near his office and bring them home for my grandmother to wear in her hair. In the evenings, they would gather at the temple in the center of town, where bells would ring loudly, fires would be lit, and the chanting of *mantras* reverberated around the temple room. Their day often started and ended this way: by connecting with devotion to the senses in the town's famous Bhadrakali temple.

These are the same rituals I have witnessed growing up, in my own home. Rituals that were repeated in my mother's home, as an Indian growing up in colonial Uganda, and in millions of homes across India and the rest of the migration patterns from there across the world. As the environments, cultures, and languages around us changed through colonization, our rituals to awaken spirit through the senses remained and passed from one generation to the next.

As a child, I grew up with my maternal grandmother. Each morning, I would sit next to her and my mother, as they offered the deities in our home temple a sensory devotion known as *pooja*. The smell of incense always permeated the air of dawn before school. I peered into the temple and wondered what deity figures represented; there were so many, some sitting poised, some standing in pairs, and others with animal friends. A ghee lamp would dance in orange flames before them. I waited eagerly, looking at the moon-colored silverware that held water, sweet raisins, cashews, and almonds as offerings I'd later get to eat, as I listened to my grandmother chant and teach me the *mantras* she opened the day and greeted the sun with.

A curious child marvels at such rituals and passes through stages of asking 'Why?' to everything. But the answers to the unquestioning devotion never seemed clear. Decades later, only after my own research into sensual living, I came to learn that the heart of these practices is not understood by the kind of rational thinking mind I was steeped in — where x happens because of y. This is a different kind of system that works with embodiment, practice, and living. It goes deeper than cognitive thinking, which has to be conscious before we are aware of it, and speaks directly to the unconscious.

By honoring the very elements we are made up of — earth, water, fire, air, and space — we honor and acknowledge the entire manifest world, including ourselves, as sacred and balanced. These elements map directly to the senses of smell, taste, sight, touch, and sound, which were all represented through the devotional offerings in our morning *pooja* ceremony when I was a child.

As I grew older, I realized that the senses offered us a way to make life itself the prayer – the piece of music that speaks directly to your soul, the taste of a ripe fruit fallen fresh from a tree, the sight of a sunset to dissolve separation from the natural world, the fragrant smell of a flower in bloom, and the touch of fresh natural water sending electricity across your skin. A life lived consciously through the senses is meditation, a prayer, a devotion, and a way of knowing the divine as it expresses itself in manifest form within and around us.

Understanding the Senses and Elements

The world, your body, and all you see around you are made up of a myriad unique compositions of the five subtle elements: earth, water, fire, air, and space. These are the subtle energies that carry their impressions of what we experience in the manifest world into our mind. We perceive them through the five senses: sight, sound, taste, touch, and smell. The gateways between the manifest world and the senses are the organs of the eyes, ears, mouth, skin, and nose, also known as the *pancha jnanendriyas*. In Sanskrit (the ancient language of the Hindu texts), *pancha* means 'five,' *jnana* means 'higher knowledge,' and *indriya* means 'an instrument to gain knowledge of the soul.'

The vehicle of the senses is the music shared between soul and spirit, which go beyond the mind. The *mahabhutas* (elements), the *tanmatras* (senses), and the *pancha jnanendriyas* (sense organs) form part of a larger structure in Tantric philosophy (something we'll be talking about later in this chapter and all throughout this book) called the *tattvas*, which form the principles of reality that constitute human experience.[1]

The *tattvas* give us a framework for understanding everything that comprises both matter and subtle energy. When we get into the more esoteric aspects of Tantra, this gives us a window onto consciousness and the very nature of the universe. It also helps us to understand how our bodies are connected to the elements in nature, as well as to qualities associated with those elements. The deeper you go into the study of the *tattvas*, you'll find that they intersect with everything from yogic philosophy to Ayurveda, an ancient Indian science of holistic health. They give us a powerful foundation for understanding that which lives in the manifest (material) world and that which resides in the unmanifest (spiritual) world – which, on closer inspection, are not as separate as we think. And the portal to understanding how they fit together lives inside our senses.

Our sense organs operate in an intricate network beyond words. Once stimulated, they communicate through the nervous system to the brain with electrochemical messages. The *sensorium* is the entire sensory apparatus of your brain, which receives, processes, and interprets sensory stimuli; it is how you convey and receive the external world, and bring it into your internal world.[2]

Our *perception* of ourselves, others, and the world comes from turning these sensory messages into thoughts. The brain receives and uses this information to work out how we respond, react, or behave. Our sense of sight tells us the difference between stepping off a curb or a cliff, and our sense of smell tells us whether something is still safe to eat. But our senses do more than keep us safe – our senses inform us about who we are and bring us into a deep connection with ourselves, others, and nature.

The Five Stages of Sensual Development

To understand where we are with our sensuality today, I have created a framework that maps different stages of our lives to our sensual development – from our earliest years and making 'sense' of the world, to the flurry of teenage hormones that often make it difficult to 'make sense' of sensuality at all. We'll explore the phases of sensual exploration, expansion, and wisdom, where our sensuality moves from a transient pleasure into a source of self-knowledge and connection to spirit – which is ultimately where this book will guide us.

Stage 1: Sensual Innocence

According to psychoanalytic theory, our personality is mostly established by the age of five. We come into the world with minds that grasp for knowledge to understand the environment around us. Before we have discovered language, we recognize the world through our senses. We are innocent, as our senses concern only ourselves and our exploration of this still-new world. Through interactions with our primary caregivers, we are given a template to understand what's happening around us that helps us to organize and make sense of our inner and outer landscape.

What we see, smell, taste, touch, and hear from our guardians, siblings, or other caregivers becomes incorporated as memories into our unconscious minds. There, it merges with and seemingly becomes our own thoughts, beliefs, and values.

Picture an iceberg that is partially visible; the majority of the iceberg lives underwater. That large underwater chunk of the iceberg is akin to the unconscious sensory processing we do in the earliest stages of life. Our sensory experiences of the world drive the formation of our personality. Early sensory experiences eventually sink into the waters of our unconscious, often driving the way we experience ourselves and interact with the world well into adulthood.

As babies, we might draw comfort from the smell of our mother, the texture of our blanket, and the colors of our home. As toddlers, we learn new words through our sensory experiences. We jump in a puddle and a parent says, 'You're all wet.' Thus, we make a connection between the water slipping down our boots and the feeling of rain drenching our clothes; now, we have a context for what 'wet' means. We also learn to use our senses to distinguish between the textures and flavors of different foods in our mouth, screaming when we don't like what we're tasting and when we crave something else. Our senses inform us when something is 'hot' or 'sharp.' It isn't until a bit later in childhood that we form stronger judgments and opinions, which is why the period of time when we are still learning primarily through our senses, rather than mental constructs around 'good' and 'bad,' is so magical.

Even when we don't have a precise or accurate memory of our early years, the purity and newness of those nascent sensory experiences can evoke a range of emotions – wonder, fear, excitement, curiosity, pleasure – that might influence us for years to come, perhaps even serving to reawaken our senses and invite us back into sensual innocence.

Stage 2: Sensual Activation

As we move from childhood into our teenage years, hormonal influences come into play. Our inward-facing exploration of the world through our senses begins to relate to others around us. We may feel a spark when we glance at our crush at school, or when we receive a glance in return. We may start to exude new pheromones, finding certain smells repulsive and others attractive. As we begin on the uncertain path of sensual connection, our innocent self-expression might be frightened into the shadows when someone calls us a 'slut' or deems what we are doing unacceptable. At this point, we start to discern for ourselves what is 'too much' and 'too little' when it comes to how far we will take our sensual exploration.

Puberty is a confusing time, to say the least, and it is filled with a host of strange and awkward sensory encounters. On the road to this change, we might be lucky enough to live in a country where some level of sex education was provided in our teenage years; in others, we might have to rely on movies, TV, media, and even pornography to explain the birds and the bees. In the Indian films I grew up watching, kissing and sex were seldom shown, but they would be alluded to as a coy married couple ran around a tree singing love ballads.

Admittedly, most 'sex education' falters in its ability to share information about sensuality, sexuality, and our changing bodies. From my experience, it usually includes information about the following:

▼ how to roll a condom onto a cucumber (and avoid getting pregnant)

▼ the many garden varieties of sexually transmitted infections you might catch by having sex, 'protected' or not

▼ the amount of water a single tampon can hold when placed in a jar

▼ what to do if you didn't heed the first two bullet points and end up in the 'unfortunate' case of teen pregnancy or catching an STI

In essence, sex education tends to be built into a busy curriculum that focuses on worst-case scenarios and fear-based instructions, instead of the things that can go right when we get up close and personal with our sensual nature in relation to another. We seldom learn about a slow, consensual approach to intimate relating with ourselves and partners. We are certainly not taught that sensuality is a practice of self-knowledge, cultivation, and personal development. We aren't encouraged to understand our bodies, their sensations, and what these sensations might mean. Knowing our desires and boundaries, as well as how to express them? Forget about it!

Please be apprised that if you, like so many others, didn't receive this information in your education, you'll absolutely receive it in this book. This is the school most of us secretly longed for but never got: the one that teaches us about the missing bridge between ourselves and sex, our sensuality.

Stage 3: Sensual Exploration

Around the time we move into adulthood, we might start to learn who we are outside of everything we've always known, the friends and family we grew up with, and the society and culture that nurtured us into being. We might start to explore our tastes and begin affirming the sensual experiences we like, such as our sense of style, favorite music, and preferred food. We might suddenly realize we like the taste of the coffee, olives, or wine, which we may not have enjoyed in our younger years.

At this stage, which occurs as we individuate and develop a stronger sense of who we are, we start to create our own sensual map — exploring our body, new lands, new partners, and new sensations. In Sanskrit, this is called *preya*, which refers to a transient pleasure that comes and goes. In some cases, we take this exploration in stride, and we are brave when it comes to making mistakes, learning, and gracefully adapting to change. Simply, we learn what we like and don't like through a series of sensory explorations with ourselves and others. For others, our culture, family, religion, or society might dissuade us from having many partners or sensual experiences — but this doesn't mean we can't develop our awareness through our own sensory interactions with the world and what is available to us. Maybe this happens through a practice that requires us to attune to our senses, such as travel, reading, dance, cooking, singing, eating, enjoying nature, listening to music, etc.

There is not always a linear trajectory or specific age range for this particular stage. Some people may not necessarily experience this period of exploration and transient pleasure in an overt way, others might stay in it their whole lives, and others will dip in and out of it, depending on their life circumstances.

Stage 4: Sensual Expansion

If you made it to this paragraph, you're probably ready for this stage. You've explored what you like and don't like but are left with a few more questions. You might be wondering: *What now? What else? What more?* You're curious to understand the sensuality within, and how you can use it to connect, love, and express yourself with rapture and aliveness. You're ready to make your life your art. You're ready to expand.

Enter... Tantra.

Etymologically, when we break down this Sanskrit word,
tan means 'to expand' and tra means 'instrument.' In
essence, Tantra gives us an instrument to expand our
consciousness and everything within it: our sensations,
our perception, and our experience of life itself.

It is also often translated as 'loom,' which is a device that weaves together cloth and tapestry. Like a loom, Tantra weaves together many different practices, from astrology and yoga to quantum physics and meditation. Its practices also weave together parts of ourselves that have been rejected, feared, or shamed. Tantra is a set of practices that can weave us back into wholeness.

It is difficult to distill Tantric philosophy into just one idea or set of ideas, as it has a multifaceted history that spans regions and time periods. With more than 64 different schools,[3] all of which will have their own approaches, each practitioner will have a different definition for Tantra. The *Tantras* also refer to a group of texts, and while their philosophy has influenced the paths of Hinduism, Jainism, Mahayana Buddhism, Chinese Taoism, and Islamic Sufism, Tantra itself is not a religion; rather, it is a mystical path that can be explored by any seeker of consciousness.

To me, Tantra is a revolutionary path for dissolving separation with the world around us and offering us a method of deep connection for knowing all of life (including others, ourselves, and our sensuality) as divine. Tantra is a powerful vehicle for sensual expansion. In expanding beyond what we know, we honor and give voice to the parts of ourselves that long to be seen and accepted; these parts often live outside of our awareness, relegated to the shadows. Tantra helps us to weave together the discarded parts of ourselves and others, which long to be acknowledged and known, so that we can experience the full spectrum of living. It's less about love and light or escapism, and more about embracing life and reality exactly as it is.

We expand in the hope that in doing so, we can transform the spark we have been searching for into a long-burning fuel to nourish us through all seasons of life.

Stage 5: Sensual Wisdom

Sensual wisdom is where we move from *avidya*, meaning 'not knowing', and return to *vidya*, or 'knowing' the bliss that lies within us. In Tantra, this bliss is known as *sukha*, a state of sweetness, joy, and ease that is everlasting because it is not tied to the material attachments we form in our lives: to a particular partner, a job, a place, a set of objects, a social status, etc. Instead, we honor our bodies as conduits of communication, and every sense organ gives us direct access to our higher power, which is everlasting bliss.

Between the earth and the skies, we treat our sensations as our sacred messengers – dissolving separation from the world around us and enhancing connection to our intuitive wisdom. It doesn't matter if the sensation is 'good' or 'bad,' because it simply exists for us to know ourselves and all of life with greater rapture.

To be in touch with our sensual wisdom is to know what our sensations are telling us. When we make the choice to respond to our sensations, we are empowered to observe and respond in a way that moves us toward connection with ourselves and the world around us.

When we don't pay attention to the wisdom of our sensations, we don't allow our true selves to be known. We do what I did early in my life: create masks behind which to move and live in the world.

Sometimes, we ignore our sensations for so long, they stop coming. The message gets left on the doorstep until it turns soggy and numb. Other times, the messengers send out a final SOS and our body finally gets the message through an alarm of pain, suffering, disease, or discomfort. In Sanskrit, this suffering is known as *dukha. Dukha* is the opposite of *sukha* and is a term found in the ancient texts known as the *Upanishads*. It relates to experiences in life that are uneasy, unpleasant, uncomfortable, or filled with difficulty, pain, and sadness.

Unfortunately, ignoring the sense messengers in our body can have great and even fatal consequences for our physical, emotional, and spiritual well-being. Opening up the doors of communication with our sensations offers us an opportunity to take in the messages they deliver, to move from dis-ease to ease and from *dukha* to *sukha*. It doesn't mean being happy all the time; rather, it is the experience of deep honesty, authenticity, and wholeness. It is the acceptance of our humanity and our divinity. This deep acceptance is what transforms sensuality from a fleeting experience into a spiritual path that takes us to our higher power and accompanies us steadily through life.

▼ Activities ▼

The Joy of the Senses

A small but powerful activity to complete at the end of each day (through visualization, meditation, or journaling) is to think of one moment related to each of the senses that brought you joy. The more you start to notice the joy of your senses, the more joy your senses will deliver to you each day.

▼ I saw...

▼ I heard...

▼ I tasted...

▼ I smelled...

▼ I touched...

Altar of the Senses

A beautiful way to honor, sharpen, and begin deepening your relationship with the senses is to create an altar space in your home. The *tattvas* we explored earlier begin with the five elements that make up the material world and feed our senses. You can bring any of the elements to your temple to remind you of the sacredness of the senses and the material world. You may use this space to begin each day or conduct the practices in this book.

Here are some examples, but you can choose any elemental aspects that feel sacred to you.

▼ earth/*prithvi* – smell: flowers, plants, crystals, soil, sand, shells, anything from nature

▼ water/*ap* – taste: a fresh cup of water, fruits, libations

- ▼ fire/*agni* - sight: a lit candle, deity sculptures/paintings, yantras (visualizations of *shakti* depicted through geometrical diagrams), representations of ancestors

- ▼ air/*vayu* - touch: a lit stick of incense, an open window, a beautifully textured fabric

- ▼ space/*akasha* - sound: singing bowls, bells, *mantras*, any sound that vibrates through space

A Portrait of the Senses

This activity has the power to deepen our awareness of, intimacy with, and appreciation for ourselves and others. You can do this activity by gazing into a mirror to grow more deeply in love with yourself through your senses. You can also do this with those around you, to get to know them even more deeply and notice things you may never have noticed before.

In this exercise, we move from seeing ourselves and others as one full physical object. By noticing with all the five senses, we gain an insight into who we/they truly are underneath. Begin by noticing yourself or another. If you are doing the practice with yourself, use a mirror. If you are doing it with another, use your mind's eye and imagine the person or let yourself be in that person's physical presence.

Notice three things about yourself or the other person, going through each sense, one by one. I have given some examples in the following exercises, but do not limit yourself to these. See what comes up when you bring your focus to yourself or the other person. You can do this by visualization or journaling.

- ▼ sight: dress style, something you/they carry, eyes, walk or posture

- ▼ sound: favorite song, a phrase often said, ringtone, voice or laugh

- ▼ taste: a favorite meal/drink, likes/dislikes, the way you/they take tea/coffee

- ▼ smell: perfume/cologne, laundry detergent, home/room

- ▼ touch: texture of clothes, hair on head/body, the feel of your/their skin

The Sense of Revelation

The senses connect us to our memories and reveal who we are. They can spark new conversations with those around us in which we can experience the same or different perceptions and learn more about how that person experiences the world. Allow the following prompts to engage you with your senses and engage others with their senses, as well.

1. Start with an observation: 'When I smell/taste/touch/hear/see X....'

2. Connect it inward: 'It makes me think of/reminds me of/makes me feel Y....'

3. Open it outward: 'What about you?'

4. Follow up: 'Where do you think that comes from?'

Example: 'When I taste Indian spices, it reminds me of my mother's, auntie's, and grandmother's cooking. It transports me right back to my childhood, where spices would fill our home before a delicious, warm meal. The taste makes me feel so at home, wherever I am in the world. Is there anything you taste that does that?'

Integration

You may wish to keep a journal for the reflection questions that you'll find at the end of each chapter.

1. Think back to each of the five stages of sensual development. What memories or reflections do you have with respect to each of these stages in your own life? How have these memories impacted the way you experience your sensuality?

2. On a scale of 1–10, how connected do you feel to your sensuality in this moment?

3. Think about the most immersive sensual experience you have had to date. What did that look or feel like? What was meaningful about it?

4. What is your intention for reading this book and moving through the practices? Use this intention as your anchor to keep you turning the pages and expanding your sensuality.

Key Takeaways

~ The five sense organs in Tantric philosophy are known as the *pancha jnanendriyas*. Among the ancients, they were revered as gateways to the soul — instruments that could help us gain knowledge of the underlying reality of the universe and our own nature.

~ Through my work, I have identified five stages of sensual development that mark the spiritual path through sensuality:

  - **Sensual Innocence:** understanding the world through our senses, which occurs in the early childhood stage

  - **Sensual Activation:** the burst of hormones during puberty that activate sensual energy within

  - **Sensual Exploration:** the transient nature of exploring pleasure through the senses, which begins in early adulthood

  - **Sensual Expansion:** sensuality beyond the bedroom as a key to fulfilled living (in this book, we use Tantra as a foundation for sensual expansion)

  - **Sensual Wisdom:** understanding sensations as sacred messengers and sensual energy that connect us to our higher power

CHAPTER 2

Knowing Your
Sensual Power (Tantra)

In this chapter, I'll share some important practices on your journey to sensuality. First, we will explore the concept of *shakti* as one of the key principles on the Tantric path, which reminds us of the innate power to heal, feel, and expand — a power that streams through all of nature and courses through our bodies, senses, and sensations.

We'll take a walk through the historical development of Tantra and discover how this path paved the way for a sensual, social, and gender revolution in thought and spiritual practices. Finally, we will look to the Tantric festival of Navaratri and practices to connect to and cultivate the divine sensual forces within.

Nine Nights of Devotion

As a child, there was a particular time of year when the smell of *saris* and *chaniya cholis* that had been sleeping through the months came to permeate the air. After school, my mother would throw open the suitcase filled with colors, and my aunties would pin yards of fabric together to drape elegantly over our bodies. My favorite of all were the skirts and blouses with tiny glistening mirrors, bonded on by frames of interweaving thread, which would deflect any remaining light as we left home under the dark sky, ready for the rituals of the night ahead.

We arrived in a hall where a warm breeze blew through vibrant, dome-shaped skirts resting on the dancing hips of the women, who moved in large swirling circles around the room. The men wore wide, flowing garments and danced amongst the women in a perfectly imperfect harmony. Each step had its own flare of personality that weaved itself through the unison of movement. I imagined that if I were a bird perched on a high tree or a star in the night sky looking down on what was happening, I'd see a mandala formation of unified, moving reds and greens, oranges washing into pinks, and whites contrasted with blacks, much like the gaze through the lens of an ever-changing kaleidoscope.

Traditional *garbi* folk music reverberated against the shining bodies, while a rhythmic sound of feet thumping and hands clapping added an extra bass to the beat. I remember so clearly the jingle of multicolored bangles and anklets shimmering across it all, the odd accessory with the fate to be lost that night crunched under the foot of a swirling dancer. I left my shoes by the thousands more at the door and said a little prayer hoping they'd still be a pair when I returned. Then, I entered the sacred ritual space where the devotional *garba* folk dance was beginning. But as I waited by my cousin's side to join in the next line of dancers – between the crisscrossing feet, bending arms, and hips that swayed from side to side – I got a glimpse of the enchanting centerpiece around which the human kaleidoscope flowed.

It was the altar.

Freshly cut flowers, leaves, and coconuts sat around it. Hundreds of tiny candles and coins cast a glowing spell. The offerings of delicious fruits and Indian sweets lay ornately placed at the feet of the sculpture that stood in the middle. From every angle of the room, it was captivating for the senses.

The figure at the center was fierce yet gentle, light in places and dark in others, dressed in beautiful new fabrics and adornments every day of the festival. It had the presence of a warrior and the caring eyes of a watchful mother, with a dagger in one hand and a lotus flower in the other. I would soon learn there were many more hands to explore of the one who smiled calmly as she sat atop a wild-maned lion. The sculpture was a personification of Goddess Durga. Alongside the thousands of people in those *garba* halls and under the open sky, there were millions around the world celebrating the festival of Navaratri: dancing, fasting, and meditating in the nine dark nights of devotion to the divine Shakti.

What Is Shakti?

In popular culture, *shakti* is sometimes very loosely translated from Sanskrit to 'divine feminine.' In the same way some words only exist in certain languages, *shakti* cannot be wholly, completely, or fully understood by this term. Rather than 'divine feminine,' which comes loaded with what society prescribes feminine to mean (usually, soft and receptive or weak and emotional), the word translates to 'power,' 'energy,' or 'matter.' (When I talk about Shakti/*shakti*, I will generally be using upper case/no italics when referring to the personification of the divine feminine manifest power and lower case/italics when referring to the general creative principle.)

Shakti is the dynamic creative force coursing through the universe, in all living beings and throughout nature.

This is so different to the limitations of 'divine feminine,' which the path of *shakti* is sometimes mixed up with. It is less to do with our gender and more to do with the power that exists within all beings. *Shakti* is the immanent aspect of the divine, meaning it's perceptible through the senses and mind. Christopher Wallis, a nondual Tantra scholar, reminds us that this means the entire manifest universe is the goddess and therefore ought to be reverenced as such. While *shakti* is personified as a goddess, along with her cosmic counterpart, the God figure Shiva (whom we will encounter later in this book), they are not actually two separate entities, but one that corresponds to two interdependent aspects of reality which represent the manifest and unmanifest world as well as power and consciousness.[1]

Shakti expresses itself in different forms. It is the storm and the calm seas, wild primal anger and love, the chair you are seated on, the book you are holding, and the words dancing across its pages. In the same way, electricity courses through the lights in your home, the networks of underground transport, and the wind turbines across the land and seas; all look different but are the same expressions of 'power,' or *shakti*.

Take a deep inhalation, and you will feel the air that fills you as *shakti* – it is the *prana*, or the electric life-force energy that streams through your body and the spark that pumps vibrations from your heart across your inner landscape. Look into a fire and see *shakti* reflected back to you in its flames as you feel the warmth of its fuel on your skin. The senses you experience from the outside and sensations you experience from the inside, including your emotions and your sensuality, are all *shakti*. *Shakti* is the dynamic creative energy of the manifest world.

The Four Shaktis

There are four distinctive types of *shakti* that will be helpful for us to understand on our explorations of sensuality as a journey not only of pleasure expansion but of discovering the innate power we have inside and around us to connect more deeply, express more freely, and take action to live with the intimacy, aliveness, and courage we desire.

1. ***Parashakti:*** This is the highest cosmic energy, whose high-generating creative power is responsible for the rotation of planets, the power of the sun and heat to create life on Earth, and the manifestation of all of existence.

2. ***Iccha shakti:*** This is the energy of free will and is associated with the individual's driving force for life. *Iccha* is desire, creative urges, ideas, longings, and wishes – and *shakti* is the power each of us has to cultivate these intentions.

3. ***Jnana shakti:*** This is the energy of knowledge and the power of the mind, whose attributes include thinking, understanding, planning, analyzing, and remembering. It is also our psychic and meditative ability to connect to higher consciousness. Both knowledge and the power of the mind help us understand how to bring our desires and will into fruition.

4. ***Kundalini shakti:*** This is both the energy of action and the power within the body, often depicted as a snake lying dormant in the pelvic bowl as sexual and sensual life force that can be cultivated, transmuted, and charged to heal our

body, expand our consciousness and creativity, and bring our desires into the manifest realm.

Tantra and the Shakti Revolution

In its formation, Tantra flipped the mainstream spiritual norm, which sought to transcend the material world in order to experience *moksha*, which translates to 'liberation' and ends the cycles of karmic rebirth. Instead of transcending everything to get to the divine, renouncing normal life and meditating in a cave, Tantra taught that the manifest world itself — including all of nature and our emotions, desires, and experiences — is the expression of divine play known as *leela*, and that we need not escape it, silence it, or demonize it. Instead, we are invited to experience it with consciousness, respect, and devotion. The world and the body itself are the temple.

Although it is argued that Tantric principles have been around since the beginning of time, across many different indigenous cultures and countries, we will look back into its codification into texts around the 6th century in India — which will help us better understand what exactly Tantra flipped and how it catalyzed revolution in society and in sensuality.

In the formation of its texts, known as the *Tantras*, this body of wisdom decided to depart from the social scale that ruled society. This scale is known as *jati*, otherwise known as India's caste system. Within this *jati* are clear and distinguishable groups known as *varnas*, or castes, each of which have set rules for life. These *varnas* are divided into four major groups: *shudra*, *vaishya*, *kshatriya*, and *brahmin*. The *shudra* caste was made up of laborers, peasants, and servants. The *vaishya* caste were the farmers, merchants, traders, and landowners. The *kshatriya* caste were the warriors and rulers. Finally, the *brahmins* were the holy caste and priests who served as an intermediary between the spiritual and human realms. But beyond these four divisions were the people who were *avarna*, meaning outside the caste system altogether. They were called *Dalits*, which literally translates to 'broken' or 'scattered.' On a practical level, their roles as street and latrine cleaners deemed them polluted, impure, and therefore 'untouchable.'

Your caste determined what you did for work, how you lived, whom you could marry, whether you could enter a temple, and even where you could drink water from. It preserved and maintained a social hierarchy. This philosophy meant that you accepted the actions known as *karmas*, which had been carried out in previous lifetimes and consequently determined the level of society you were born into during this life.

If you were born into a particular caste, the only way to elevate yourself was through an arduous life of good *karmas*, which pertained to fulfilling one's duty, known as *dharma*. *Dharma* was always dependent on one's caste. One could not simply work harder or study to become a priest, share spiritual teachings, or manage a temple – one had to be born *brahmin*, and more importantly, one had to be born male.[2]

In the 6th century, an opportunity for change emerged. Up until that point, spiritual knowledge was passed down through *sruti*. This translates to 'that which is heard' and was the way spiritual knowledge got passed through an oral tradition for those socially elevated enough to hear it.

Then, the revolutionary series of texts known as the *Tantras* emerged. These are believed to have originated among the ascetic and outcaste groups that lived on the margins of society, often around the cremation grounds. These texts presented a promise of power for both the lover and warrior, the merchant and servant, the woman and street sweeper. They offered hope and regeneration in the face of systemic oppression and turned the caste system on its head.

According to the 7th century Svacchanda Tantra, 'All those who have been initiated are of equal nature. Once a person has taken up the Tantric system, they may never mention their former caste.'[3]

The wisdom once passed from the hands of the fair few was bestowed through Tantra to open a spiritual path for all in society. It became known as a path for the everyday householder. Up until this point, society had focused on climbing up the rungs of the *varnas*, which could only be achieved over several lifetimes, if at all. But now, it was time to go deep down into the darkness from where we emerged.

From the head, Tantra invited us to move into the body. From the crown, symbolizing the motivation to climb castes to higher consciousness and leave behind sexuality, we were asked to look down to the chalice of our roots and the power of our manifest sensations and sexual energy. The understanding of our very own essence would bring spiritual evolution and access to lasting *sukha* and spiritual bliss. Plus, we didn't have to wait for the next lifetime — it could be experienced right here and right now. The key to our power was returned to the alchemy of the inner world with doctrines and rituals to move us away from the hierarchal structure and into the all-pervasive *shakti* that existed within all beings.

On this earthly plane, *shakti* as a creative, dynamic force was most tangible through the birth of babies. The female bodies that were once seen as an impediment to spiritual growth were now revered for having particular strengths, including a naturally occurring connection to *shakti*. For the first time, initiation, participation, and sharing of spiritual practices and rituals were open to women. For this reason, and given the time in which these texts were written, *shakti* became known as a primordial 'female' energy because it is the creative power that births the manifest world. This is why it is sometimes called the 'divine feminine.'

> Shakti *and creative potential exist in all beings, whether we give birth or not. We all hold creative potential: We can make art, birth ideas, nurture our hearts, be with our sensations, love our children, tend to our lands, and nourish others. Tantra invites us to give deep respect to the* shakti *that was lost, oppressed, and pillaged through years of patriarchy, war, and colonialism.*

It invites us to get closer to *shakti* in ourselves, through ritual, *mantras*, meditation, embodiment, and also a deep reverence for women, wives, mothers, grandmothers, sisters, cousins and friends. Tantra honors the *shakti* within our queer community and the *shakti* that has been oppressed in men. Tantra honors the *shakti* of the natural world, too, our planet, oceans, animals, and plants, with the same devotion.

It's said that the path to healing ourselves and the world can be found by healing our relationship with *shakti* within. Tantra's freeing approach created a way to explore the dynamic forces of gender, energy, and expansion beyond labels, as we will continue to discover.

The universal power and energy that is invisible to the naked eye yet pulsing through the manifest world took ascetics a lifetime to meditate on and understand. To offer a more accessible understanding of this power to the everyday householder, *shakti* was given a visual personification as a goddess with many different forms and faces, often referred to as Parvati, Durga, and Kali, among many other names. These were not deities higher than us or outside of ourselves, but ways to realize, remember, and recognize the different ways *shakti* flows through each of us through its archetypes.

Tantra, in its own revolutionary ways, returned us to knowing that we're powerful, multidimensional beings birthed from the energy of the manifest world that is Shakti herself.

Shakti Rediscovered

I was in my early twenties when Shakti called me back to her shores. I remember looking through the window of my crooked apartment in Beijing; it was dark in the kind of winter that would chap your skin if you stayed in its winds too long. I lived on the fifth floor, in a building with unending flights of stairs — the kind that stole your breath and made you sweat before freezing you over with the drafts from its broken windows.

It had been some years since I'd first chosen to move from my dancing heart to a dizzy head filled with the rules and regulations of a legal career. I stood in the kitchen with the lights switched off, looking at the metal bars on my window. For a split second, I questioned whether they were intended to keep people from climbing in or from jumping out. In a big, busy city full of tall buildings, there was plenty of shade for dark thoughts. I turned my eyes from the bars back to the window, catching sight of myself in the reflection: an empty black silhouette standing behind silver bars.

In that moment, a force – much like the one that had danced me for those nine long divine nights – came through me, and my hand reached for the kitchen drawer. I skimmed over the knives and onto the next surface, where I pulled open my camera and took a picture. I noticed that when I looked down at the picture I'd taken, there was something different looking back. Up until that moment, I could only see the black empty figure, but now there was a twinkling of city lights cascading in the reflection, from my heart right down to my pelvis, where it sparkled with the first twinge of life I'd experienced in a very long time.

That surge of inspiration that struck me in the dark kitchen was Shakti herself. The picture sent a bolt of electricity through the nerves I thought had died when a Google search couldn't answer: 'Why is my pelvis numb?' It showed me an alarming geographical pinpoint where I needed to look next. I was encouraged to follow the lights in the picture, starting with the cage I'd kept around my heart and pelvis, which had forced me to live in my head. There was an ocean of sensual forces stuck in this high-walled dam I had built between my mind and my body. Slowly, a trickle of sensual life force started to drift through the cracks. Having lived with no signs, no sensations, no emotions, for a series of long winters, this felt huge.

I picked up a pen and started to write again. It felt like the first piece of bread broken after a long, hungry day of fasting. I caught the first spoke of sun peeking through the curtains in the morning; the pink blossoms lined the path to spring, and the drafts of warm breeze flowed through my hair as I cycled with no destination on the last day of that corporate job with the office in the sky.

Navaratri Rediscovered

Although we had been attending the festival of Navaratri and paying homage to Shakti through my ancestral lineage for generations and lifetimes beyond remembering, no one around me could answer some of the deeper-rooted questions I was asking when I set off to explore sensuality and the origin of these traditions. However, I had a deep feeling that I wanted to get to know her, the one who came to find me in my darkest days and call me back to her sensual shores.

I returned to India, the land of my family and ancestors. I spent subsequent years of exploration in Asia, sitting with wise medicine women and monks, gurus and *sanyasins* (devotees), philosophy teachers and spiritual guides. I sat in deep, silent meditations and loud, dynamic catharsis. I climbed mountains to reach divine Tantric temples and meet the mystics who would share with me their ancient path and its practices.

I learned more about this festival of Navaratri I so loved. *Nava* translates to 'nine,' and *ratri* translates to 'nights.' While most festivals around the world are celebrated during the day, this one embodies the sacredness of the darkest night sky, which belongs to Shakti. The dancing, swirling circles of the *garba* folk dance come from the Sanskrit *garbha*, meaning 'womb,' and the kaleidoscope of merging colors was actually a representation of that womb whose center represents the power of creation.

Before deities and sculptures depicted Shakti through the great goddess Durga, a lantern known as the *garbha deep* was placed at the center to represent the powerful divine forces of the womb, around which the room spun. Barefoot, the dancers kissed the mother of all beings with their devotional dance; the long, repetitive movements that pounded the ground evoked the *kundalini shakti* in the body. When a lot of people come together to invoke *shakti*, it nourishes them but also affects the collective consciousness and makes it easier for that energy to show up in the world.

As I encountered more and more spiritual paths in my travels, I further distinguished Tantra as one of the only ones that held the manifest world and all aspects within it, including our sensuality and bodily sensations, as deeply revered and sacred.

Kundalini shakti, as we explored earlier in this chapter, is the sexual life force that lives in the pelvis. When it releases, it traverses the body and transforms into sensual energy that can heal us, empower us, and spark deep insights and creativity. In the Tantra Yoga and traditional Kundalini Yoga traditions, this energy is visualized as a snake and coaxed up the spine through a series of *asanas* (movement and postures), *mantras* (chanting as an instrument for the mind), *pranayama* (cultivation of life force, often through practices with the breath), *bandhas* (physical, psychic, and energetic locks), *yantras* (visualizations of *shakti* depicted through geometrical diagrams), *pooja* (devotional ceremonies), and meditations on the deity figures.

During Navaratri, the four types of *shakti* are awakened and serve as a reminder of the power we have to connect the *parashakti* of cosmic energy, *iccha shakti* of free will, *jnana shakti* of knowledge, and *kundalini shakti* to take dynamic action within.

Tantra maps four Navaratris through the year that invite us to tune in to the rhythms of nature, change our seasonal routines, and charge up our power and strength. Not all Navaratris look the same; for example, the Navaratri that shares the *garba* folk dance usually occurs during the biggest Navaratri celebration, known as the *Sharadiya* or Autumn Navaratri.

The four Navaratris are roughly during the following months, though they depend on the lunar calendar:

▼ **Sharadiya Navaratri** – Autumn Navaratri (the most well-known, around October/November)

▼ **Magha Navaratri** – Winter Navaratri (sometimes called *Gupta* or Secret Navaratri, around January/February)

▼ **Chaitra Navaratri** – Spring Navaratri (the second most well-known, around March/April)

▼ **Ashadha Navaratri** – Monsoon Navaratri (sometimes called *Gupta* or Secret Navaratri, around June/July)

The Origins of Navaratri

The festival of Navaratri includes a mythological story that comes from a sacred devotional text called the Devi Mahatmyam, from around 600 CE. It marks a significant change and places *shakti* as the key source of power and spiritual development. The name of the text translates from Sanskrit as the 'Glory of the Goddess.' I share the myth from the text here to connect to the powerful source that placed *shakti*, our sensations, and our sensuality at the forefront of spirituality.

I hope that sharing its mythological origins provides an opportunity to give context and pay homage to the roots of Tantra, which are often forgotten. Mythology isn't so much about if it is true or really happened, but about if any part of the story is true for you. Deities come alive when their characteristics are invoked within us. They transform from a figure in a myth into a palpable energy, archetype, or universal power. You will explore the *Nava Durgas*, or the nine goddesses of Navaratri, in the practice at the end of this chapter.

The Crushing of Mahishasura

Once, there was a buffalo demon named Mahishasura. He was often losing fights with the *devas*, or gods. He held this begrudgingly in his mind and promised his father that he'd become the most powerful being in all of creation – and that he would beat the *devas*. He began his *tapasya*, a regimen of strict fasting and chanting sacred prayers to gain spiritual powers. After years of practice, Brahma, the creator god, granted him the boon of invincibility against humans and *devas*. Mahishasura began to spread his evil intention among humans on Earth before ascending to do the same in the heavens.

The boon Mahishasura had been granted meant he could not be defeated by humans or *devas*. He was confident that with his size and strength, no goddesses (known as *devis*) would be able to take him on, so he had omitted them from his request.

The gods were helpless and were left wandering, with no hope of using their powers for a number of years. After some thought, Vishnu, the god of preservation, found a loophole. The *devas* put their strength together and came into a deep *dhyana* (concentration), as their thoughts, consciousness, and intentions formed to call forth the feminine force that would beat the demon. The strength of their intention was fruitful, and soon, a large fire appeared in the sky. From it, the goddess Durga, who would vanquish Mahishasura, appeared.

In each of her hands, she held the tools that would help slay the demon. She carried the *chakra* (discus) of Vishnu, the trident of Shiva, and a pot of the holy waters from the River Ganges from Brahma. Varun, the god of the water, gave lotus flowers and a loud ringing conch that could be heard across all the ages. Vayu, the god of the winds, gave her a bow and a never-ending supply of arrows. Indra, the king of the gods, offered his thunderbolt. Vishwakarma, the divine architect of the gods, gave the axe; Yama, god of death, a staff; and Kuber, god of wealth, a cup of wine. Surya, the sun god, gave his blinding rays; Tvasta, the artisan god, gave her a divine mace; and finally, Himavat, god of the mountains, presented her with a lion to ride on. Regardless of the tools, only the *shakti* within her could slay the demon.

Mahishasura caught wind of this and tried to play tricks, transforming into a handsome man to try and get her to marry him. But Durga cut through his charm with one firm breath, and her own army appeared. Their battle went on for nine nights, until finally, Durga won the battle and released the world from the suffering it had so long endured. All the *devas* thanked Durga, leaving the all-pervasive power of the world, known as *shakti*, in her hands.

Your Own Navaratri

In each of the nine divine nights of Navaratri, Durga transforms into different *avatars* with unique powers to beat the demon Mahishasura. An *avatar* is a manifestation of a deity with its own unique characteristics. The 'tri' of Navaratri refers to the three aspects of Shakti, or the divine feminine aspects of reality: Goddess Kali, Goddess Lakshmi, and Goddess Saraswati. Each of these goddesses can be divided into three more goddesses, making up the nine faces of Durga. Each *avatar* reflects back to us a unique power of our own to explore, cultivate, harness, and charge the *shakti* within. They gift us their powers, manifest insight, and transform the lives of their followers.

You may choose to celebrate your own Navaratri by exploring the archetypes of each goddess, or by carving out time to dive deeper into your sensual and spiritual development during one of the four Navaratris. You can also choose to join us at SOSA for our annual celebrations for the *Sharadiya Navaratri*, the final Navaratri of the year, online.

Goddess Kali — Endings and Beginnings

▼ **Day 1: *Shailaputri*** — Self-determination: Break away from habits and patterns; make space in your diary for the festival to focus on self-care and spiritual/sensual practices; evaluate and set an intention.

▼ **Day 2: *Brahmacharini*** — Self-discipline: Connect to your determination, distilling the voice of others and the inner critic from your own; use activities to connect to your willpower, such as fasting, ice bathing, and yoga.

▼ **Day 3: *Chandraganta*** — Authentic power: Connect to your inner power by looking at where your power may be resting in attachments, dependency, or external validation; look at where you could set boundaries to protect and harness your power. This might look like creating boundaries around screen time, not checking work emails after a certain hour, canceling plans or subscriptions, etc.

Goddess Lakshmi — Pleasure, Wealth, and Beauty

▼ **Day 4: *Kushmanda*** — True happiness: Connect to joy and pleasure through activities, people, and places that bring you happiness. Notice how it feels to smile.

▼ **Day 5: *Skandamata*** — Self-love: Connect to care, nourishment, and inner kindness with self-massage, gifting yourself, and making contact with Earth and nature. Explore your relationship with your mother and the mother within.

▼ **Day 6: *Katyayani*** — Manifestation: Connect to your creative ideas and dreams; make a plan of action to bring these dreams to life.

Goddess Saraswati — Creativity and Flow

▼ **Day 7: *Kalaratri*** — Embracing darkness: Connect to what you've been avoiding, which could be something practical, like a task or your taxes, or emotional, like a particular experience or conversation. Don't be afraid to reach out for support to a friend or therapist.

▼ **Day 8: *Mahagauri*** — Rebirth and play: Connect to your inner child by writing a letter to them, asking them what they need, and responding with what you felt you could have had more/less of as a child; offer yourself that today or connect with a playful 'new' activity.

▼ **Day 9: *Siddhidatri*** — Transformation: Acknowledge your unique gifts and plan to use them; steer away from self-doubt and take time to truly see the talents, skills, and light within through journaling and setting time over the next season to nourish these aspects within yourself.

Day 10 is Dussehra, which represents victory. This closes the nine nights of Navaratri with a night of celebration. We harness the hard work done over the past nine nights. Dussehra is an auspicious day to start any new ventures, projects, habits, and actions for the season ahead.

Charge Up the Shakti Within

Now that we know her origins, it's time to meet Shakti within. This is a power that can be cultivated to empower ourselves; to clear blocks; and to energize, harmonize, and connect to the sacred messengers she carries through our body in the form of our senses and sensations.

Like personal and spiritual growth, sensual growth takes practice; you'll start to feel Shakti as you consistently devote yourself to her presence inside your body. She will empower any practice you do — whether that is your movement practice, a creative project, a master's degree, a job, or any of your other dreams. Shakti will enrich your senses so that sound, touch, taste, smell, and sight are experienced with a deep joy, aliveness, and fulfilment. This will flower into your relationships, sensuality, and pleasure, so that you form deeper connections with life itself.

Here are some practices for you to connect to and charge up your inner *shakti*.

▼ Activities ▼

Fill Your Sensual Cup

There are three diaphragms in the body: the respiratory diaphragm in the chest, laryngeal diaphragm in the throat, and pelvic diaphragm in the pelvis. Many practices only invite us to breathe into the chest and lungs. The chest expands as we inhale and depresses as we exhale. The pelvic floor lengthens and travels outward as we inhale and travels back up to its original position as we exhale. Tantra yoga invites us to bring awareness to the pelvic diaphragm (in the pelvis) in order to connect with the *shakti* that naturally resides there. Here are the instructions for this practice:

1. Sit comfortably.

2. Begin to bring attention to your breath.

3. Notice how your breath moves your throat, chest, and pelvic floor (expanding and relaxing as you inhale, contracting as you exhale). Don't change anything – just watch. It may not automatically relax, as we can hold tension here.

4. Keep practicing and sending the instruction that it's safe to let go and relax.

5. After some time, you can also consciously inhale and expand the pelvic floor, then exhale, imagining there are strings tied between the two sit bones, which draw together as you exhale.

6. You can also practice isolating the different muscles: for example, inhaling and expanding to relax, and exhaling to contract the perineum (the area between the anus and the genitals). You can do the same with the urethra. To feel this part of your body, you can imagine stopping the flow of excrement or urine.

7. Try doing all of the above separately and then at the same time; at first, everything might move together at once. Your *shakti* muscles are in training, and in time, your neural pathways will connect to send oxygenated, nutrient-rich blood to the areas to enhance sensation and energetic flow.

8. Remember, relaxing is important for releasing tension we may be holding in our body. Don't be afraid to make sounds and exhale from your mouth as you release.

Sufi Swirls

1. Sit comfortably on a seat or with your legs crossed. Place your hands on your knees, relax your shoulders, and take note of how you are feeling before the practice.

2. Take a few breaths to arrive in your body. Tune in to your pelvis and ground your sit bones into the earth.

3. Start to move your upper body in circles, starting smaller and then getting bigger.

4. Once you have found a rhythm with your movement, find a rhythm with your breath.

5. Inhale as you expand, and exhale as you compress.

6. Once you have found a rhythm with your breath, move your attention to your pelvic floor.

7. As you inhale and expand your breath, relax your pelvic floor. As you exhale, lift and squeeze your pelvic floor.

8. Continue to squeeze and relax your pelvic floor as you swirl.

9. Come into stillness and observe the sensations. As you pause, breathe and explore visualizing or 'transmuting' the *shakti* energy, moving it into different areas of the body you would like to share its nourishment, healing, and power with.

10. Repeat steps 3-9, moving your body in circles of the opposite direction.

Cakki Calanasana (Mill Churning Pose)

1. Sit on the ground with your legs as wide apart as feels comfortable. If your knees stay bent, sit on a cushion and roll a blanket or place pillows underneath your knees.

2. Take a few breaths to arrive in your body. Tune in to your pelvis and ground your sit bones into the earth.

3. Interlace your fingers and stretch your arms out in front of you at shoulder height.

4. Lean forward and start to draw circles, moving from one foot back toward yourself, and to the other foot and back again.

5. Find your rhythm with your movement and then with your breath; inhale as you move forward and exhale as you draw back.

6. Once you have found a rhythm with your breath, move your attention to your pelvic floor.

7. As you move forward, inhale and relax your pelvic floor; as you exhale, move back, squeezing your pelvic floor.

8. Come into stillness and observe the sensations. As you pause, breathe and explore visualizing or 'transmuting' the *shakti* energy, moving it into different areas of the body you would like to share its nourishment, healing, and power with.

9. Repeat steps 3-9, moving your body in circles of the opposite direction.

Shakti Mudra

A *mudra* is a yogic hand gesture that connects the energetic channels in the body to redirect energy back into specific areas of the body. *Shakti mudra* redirects energy back into *Svadhistana chakra* (the second *chakra*) and the pelvis, helping us to connect to creativity, sensuality, emotions, and passion.

1. Find a comfortable seat, place your hands on your thighs with palms facing upward, and take a few breaths to arrive.

2. Bend your thumbs to touch the palms.

3. Wrap the index and middle finger around the thumb.

4. Bring both your hands together to touch the tips of the ring fingers and little fingers with the other hand.

5. The knuckles of your middle and index finger should also be touching.

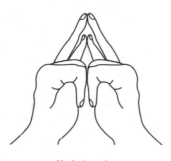

Shakti mudra

6. Hold the gesture near your pelvis or heart while you meditate.

Options: Chant *vam* or *om*, while standing/sitting after *asana* or *pranayama* practice.

The Shakti Flow

1. Start in tabletop pose on a yoga mat, or on a soft, supported surface for your knees, with your hands under your shoulders, your knees under your hips, and the top of your feet flat on the earth or toes tucked under.

2. As you inhale, arch your spine, shine your heart forward, lift your chin to stretch your throat, relax your jaw, soften your belly to the earth, lift your tailbone to the sky, and relax your pelvic floor.

3. As you exhale, press your hands and feet into the earth, round your spine, tuck your chin, draw your navel in toward your spine, tuck your pelvis and gently squeeze the pelvic floor.

4. Repeat Steps 2 and 3, going back and forth between these motions: inhaling, relaxing, expanding, exhaling, contracting. Slow for relaxing, and quicken for activating.

5. For Circles and Eights, step the hands further forward beyond the shoulders.

6. Circle the hips in one direction and then the opposite.

7. Create figure-eight motions between the back of your mat and your hands.

8. Roll the *shakti* energy along your spine in an undulating movement.

9. Forget any shape and move freely, expressing primally how the body wants to move and express itself.

10. Play with breath and stillness between each of the transitions.

Move, Dance, and Flow

The feet and pelvis are intimately connected through the fascia and offer a great way to evoke *shakti*. Any movement that involves the feet bouncing on the ground will help evoke it. Some examples are skipping, running, trampolining, *garba* dance during *Sharadiya Navaratri*, belly dancing, hula-hooping, twerking, and shaking. You can also stretch the toes and arches of the feet. In our online Tantra Yoga community, we have a Shakti Flow class each week, which takes traditional rigid *hatha* postures and adds more circular, flowing movements, so that *shakti* energy can flow through the body, with deep awareness of the pelvic region.

Integration

1. How is Shakti, or the 'divine feminine,' represented within your own cultural lineage, religion, or upbringing?

2. In the story about the Goddess Durga defeating the demon Mahishasura, what did the demon, the battle, and Durga represent for you? Was there any other part of the myth that resonated?

3. After you do each of the practices in this chapter, describe the sensations in your body. Journal about it. Notice how your sensations change over time. Does working with the pelvic floor bring up any images or memories? Be gentle as you explore this.

4. Reflect on what you learned about Navaratri. Look up and add the four seasonal Navaratris to your diary to celebrate nine nights for connecting back to your *shakti* and sensual power.

KEY TAKEAWAYS

~ *Shakti* is power, energy, matter, and the dynamic creative force of the universe. Rather than relating to a gender, it is an energy that exists within all beings and through nature.

~ The four *shaktis* are: *parashakti* (cosmic energy), *iccha shakti* (energy of desire, creative urges, ideas, longings, and wishes), *jnana shakti* (energy of knowledge and the power of the mind), and *kundalini shakti* (the energy of action and sensual/sexual life force).

~ Tantra emerged as a revolutionary path for social equality across gender, class, sexuality, and race.

~ The festival of Navaratri occurs seasonally and is made up of nine nights of honoring the different faces of Shakti, as well as evoking them within.

~ You can work with a series of practical physical exercises that charge the *shakti* within.

CHAPTER 3

Knowing Your
Sensual Cycle (Ayurveda)

In this chapter, we'll move further into the sister sciences of Tantra, Ayurveda, and Yoga to deepen our sensuality, not only through the seasons but also more intricately: through the body, during the month, and throughout our life.

In understanding our sensual cycle, we come to understand that our different states and stages of life are precious and full of wisdom. We don't chase sensuality or expect it to feel the same every day. We'll look at the different approaches to the menstrual and sensual cycle from the Ayurvedic and Tantric traditions. We'll examine the different sensual zones mapped to the moon cycle in ancient texts. We'll use this inspiration to track the sensual cycle to six phases, which will indicate to us the best time to undertake particular tasks, as well as reveal when we are most and least sensual. These are not only relevant for menstruators but for every being — because every being is cyclical.

A Return to Cyclical Living

Wrapped up in a cocoon of shame and fear of getting pregnant, I spent more than 10 years on and off various contraceptive methods. From the age of 13, my friends and I had gone from popping candies to popping contraceptive pills. I had begun by taking a pill to delay my period before going on a school water-sports holiday in the Ardèche, France. Friends around me were on the pill to treat acne, cramps, and other hormonal 'imbalances.' It seemed for any of the hormonal changes we were going through, it was commonplace for our doctor to prescribe a contraceptive pill.

Lacking any real menstrual education, I was put onto as many pills as colors you'd find in a Smarties box: ones that made my boobs big and bouncy, ones that made them small and saggy, ones that gave me spots, ones that made me aroused, ones that made me feel crazy, ones that made me numb. Then, there were the ones I accidentally missed taking. Those ones had me on my knees praying for my period that month. The whole cycle was spent running in circles, making every effort to chase my period away and then hoping it would arrive again to confirm I wasn't pregnant. Menstruation, I thought, was a huge inconvenience, beyond my control.

The copper coil gave me 10-day periods with pain so debilitating I could no longer walk, move, or think. I took time off work, which my manager gave me without question as soon as I so much as mentioned the 'p' word. I cried to the doctor after a year and pleaded that they take it out. They did, before putting another one up there – this time, a hormonal coil that stopped my period completely for five years.

While my body was no longer reproductive, those five years were the most 'productive' I'd ever been. I could work around the clock,

24/7, 365 days a year, and have very few or no fluctuations in my physical or emotional state each month. That meant spending less money on menstrual products and gaining more time. I saved 12 weeks a year, three months where I could work when other bleeders might not have. Perfect for a career in law and traveling with more room in my backpack. I ran a 0.02 percent risk of pregnancy and a 99.98 percent lack of understanding about the unique power of the menstrual cycle.

As I returned to the practices of my ancestors, the three sister sciences of Tantra, Ayurveda, and Yoga gathered in a circle around me. Like siblings welcoming home a sister who had gone astray, each had their own unique character and would, piece by piece, share with me the wellspring of wisdom, energy, intuition, creativity, and connection that are available when we follow our cyclical rhythms.

When my period returned after taking out the coil, it felt like it was my first time again. Instead of feeling muddled with confusion and hiding pads up my sleeve, I went to my teacher for a *pooja*, another devotional ceremony. As the *pooja* began, my teacher offered devotion to the dynamic forces of *shakti* that were residing in me through my cycle.

My teacher offered a beautifully fragrant sandalwood paste (representing the earth element) to my forehead, placed fruit at my feet (representing the water element), circled a ghee lamp around my face three times (representing the fire element), circled incense around me three times (representing the air element), and rang loud bells (representing the space element). When he placed the cooling sandalwood paste and a red *kumkum* powder on my forehead and crown, something came alive. The *kumkum* powder, a vermilion paste, anointed my third eye in the same color as the blood I was bleeding. It sent tears rolling down my face, which trickled down my neck and landed between my breasts, anointing my heart.

I felt the embodiment of the goddess figures I grew up seeing in the temples. It seemed I had been offered an opportunity to rewrite the narrative in my body and through my senses around menstruating. What was once filled with shame, pain, and inconvenience became sacred. Instead of an enemy I chased away, it became a welcomed wise elder who visited me each month, bestowing invaluable intel for me to follow on the operation of my body, mind, spirit, and purpose – if only I took the time to listen.

In my teens, I thought my menstrual cycle marked me a grown woman, but with this knowledge, my cycle marked me a grown goddess.

Ayurveda and Approaches to Cyclical Living

At the change of every season, the trees change colors, undress, stand naked, and then get dressed again. The temperatures rise and fall. Animals mate in some months and in others move into hibernation. Each cycle, the moon opens to brighten the skies, and then waxes and wanes into darkness again. Each day, the sun rises, nourishes life on Earth, and sets again. Such is the changing, dynamic nature of the manifest world and its *shakti*. It is only we unfortunate humans who have set upon each other and ourselves the expectation to turn up in our work, relationships, and sensuality the same way 365 days a year.

Ayurveda means 'knowledge of life' and is an ancient healing science and medical system based on living in balance and harmony with the internal and external natural world. This school is inextricably linked with its sister sciences, Tantra and Yoga, something that is often forgotten in the Western ways of practicing these ancient traditions. According to Dr. Vasant Lad, Ayurvedic practitioner and professor, Ayurveda is the foundation, Yoga is the body, and Tantra is the head. They form an interdependent trinity, which means our optimal physical, emotional, and spiritual health depend on the practice of all three.

Ayurveda recognizes the huge environmental shifts that take place each season. It encourages us to build daily regimens known as *dina chariya* and seasonal regimens known as *ritu chariya* to support the mind, body, and spirit while we transition through the year. For this reason, Navaratri comes around four times annually, in different shapes and forms, to invite us to connect back to our *shakti*, support the homeostasis of our body, and help us to transition through the change of our external environment to maintain optimal balance.

Homeostasis is the self-regulating process by which any organism maintains stability while adjusting to the conditions that are best for its survival. In Ayurveda, this optimal balance is called our *prakriti* – translating to our 'original' or 'true' nature. We are born into the world with our *prakriti* and tasked with the role of looking after it in our body.

Our *prakriti* is made up of the five elements that are present in nature and in the human body. These five elements combine and coordinate to form the three *doshas*, or the governing forces found throughout nature, the seasons, the times of the day, and within the functioning of our bodies. Each person has a certain body composition made up of the elements. The three doshas are:

▼ *vata*: air and space

▼ *pitta:* fire and water

▼ *kapha:* earth and water

When the *doshas* are in balance, we are close to our true nature; when they are out of balance, we are in our *vikruti*. It's similar to when the temperature increases in the atmosphere and we start to see imbalances in other areas, such as heavier rainfall, floods, droughts, and melting icebergs. As the elements change, so does the world – and as the world changes, so do we. Therefore, to harmonize the internal world, Ayurveda and Tantra work with natural cycles to teach us to adapt to the body's needs and functions, which are also changing, depending on external influences. It might be the season we are experiencing, the time of day, or our age in the cycle of life (see the table at the end of the chapter).

Our *prakriti* is derived from conception and birth, and is influenced by the genetic lineages of our parents. Our *vikruti* stems from an imbalance or predominance of a particular *dosha*, which is influenced by lifestyle and experiences. There are three significant causes of imbalance, disease, and disconnection from our true nature or optimal balance. These include a low digestive strength (*agni*, which translates to 'fire,' and is another name for this digestive force in the body), the suppression of natural urges (such as belching, burping, sleep, urination, ejaculation, etc.), and finally, the change of the seasons, when many of us experience lower immunity, influenza, colds, and changes in mood.

It makes sense – it's hard to feel our sensuality when we are constipated, ill, or tired. This is why what we eat, how we move, how we express our natural urges (which are often suppressed in society), and how we adapt our daily, seasonal, and lifespan regimens are important. This is a reminder to burp like my aunties in India – it's only natural! Various points through the year, such as Navaratri or the solstices and equinoxes, provide us incredible opportunities to support this internal balance from which we can experience deeper sensuality in each season.

You can find out your *prakriti dosha* by consulting with an Ayurvedic practitioner; there is also a *dosha* quiz on the SOSA website (*see p.xxi*). When you know your *dosha*, you can empower yourself with knowledge about how to return to your true nature and take specific actions to support and nourish your unique composition.

You are not the same as everyone around you. Your journey to deeper sensuality is unique. It's important to take a holistic approach to maintaining your prakriti, *staying close to your true* shakti *nature, and knowing what to do when you move away from it.*

You may notice your entire lifestyle transform when you do this. From this place of inner balance you will experience the deepest connection, sensuality, and aliveness.

You can work with the three *doshas* and their associated elements to find ways to balance your energy based on where you are in your menstrual cycle or life phase.

Vata

Elements: Air and space

Force: Moving force that extracts nutrients and expels waste

Body: Pelvic region, colon, bladder, urinary tract, legs, arms, bones, nervous system, and mind

Menstrual phase: Menstruation; downward flow to move blood out of the body

For balance: Go inward with rest, essential oils, meditation, restorative yoga, journaling, and grounding touch

Life phase: Age 50+, the time of wisdom when the body becomes lighter, thinner, and drier

Pitta

Elements: Fire and water

Force: Force that processes and transforms

Body: Stomach, small intestine, umbilical, sweat, blood, and lymph glands

Menstrual phase: Secretory; progesterone rises with a shift from ovulation to premenstrual

For balance: Plan alone time with gentle movement and slow yoga, a balanced diet, fluid touch, and massage with oils

Life phase: Ages 17–50, the time when the inner fire is needed to work, be active, and have a family if you choose

Kapha

Elements: Earth and water

Force: Force that holds everything together

Body: Head, neck, chest, thorax, joints, fat, and tissues

Menstrual phase: Proliferative; estrogen rises with a shift from the end of menstruation to ovulation

For balance: Plan social connection with higher energy, stronger movement, and yoga

Life phase: Ages 0–16, the time of growth, when *kapha* is the predominant force

The Five Winds

All the sister sciences honor cyclical wisdom to empower the way we live through each month. We do not show up the same each day of the month, but are impacted by fluctuating energy, moods, and even sensuality.

According to Ayurveda, there are five *vayus* ('winds' in Sanskrit) that govern different areas of the body and perform different functions that influence physical and emotional health. These are energetic forces that move in specific directions, with the task of overseeing different bodily functions while operating in harmony together.

▼ *Prana vayu* translates as 'forward-moving air' and is located at the heart. The flow is inward and upward, and is responsible for the way we receive the world, and how we nourish our senses and thoughts.

▼ *Apana vayu* translates as 'the air that moves away' and is located in the pelvic floor and lower abdomen. The flow is downward and out, and is responsible for reproduction and elimination in the body.

▼ *Udana vayu* translates to 'that which carries upward' and is located in the throat. The flow is circular around the head and neck, and is responsible for holding us up and governing speech.

▼ *Samana vayu* translates to 'the balancing air' and is located in the navel. The flow is from the outside of the body to the center, and is responsible for digestion of everything from food and air to emotions, thoughts, and experiences.

▼ *Vyana vayu* translates as 'outward moving air' and is located across the whole body. The flow is from the center of the body to the outside, and is responsible for the circulation of everything and assisting the other *vayus*.

When we are menstruating, the *apana vayu* is doing its work to eliminate. The body is in its phase of dissolution. The incredible book *Rtu Vidya*, by Sinu Joseph,[1] explores the ancient science behind indigenous menstruation practices in India. Joseph shares how this means that the body has been gifted a period not only to dispel physical toxins and residues from food and chemicals in the physical layer of the body, but also to release the mental, energetic, and emotional toxins we have accumulated over the month's cycle.

Activities such as *pranayama* and inversions, chanting, or visiting a temple nourish the body's *udana vayu* and upward-facing winds, which are contraindicative to the primary task of downward elimination in the body at this time. Traditionally, menstruators are invited to see this period of dissolution as a gift to rest, rejuvenate, and connect to the heightened *shakti* wisdom within their body, as it is considered a temple charged with high spirit and the forces of nature.

Indigenous traditions do not only see the menstrual cycle as useful for those who would like to get pregnant and an inconvenience for those who don't. Instead, any 'body' who aligns with their cyclical nature is provided with the opportunity to receive a 'monthly report.' The consistency, color, smell, and duration of discharge and menstrual blood are all indicators of the whole body's functions, and can give us information about imbalances or potential diseases. The changing levels of energy, social interaction, motivation, desire, and sensuality can be tracked to help us connect with a report from the body's inner physician and wisdom, and to empower our monthly cycles.

The Sensual Cycle

I was in a menstrual cycle training with the wonderful Uma Dinsmore-Tuli a few years ago and came across an inspiring fellow student. She was calm yet fierce, confident yet collected, and she piqued my curiosity as she shared her post-menopause experiences.

As the training went on, she shared how, contrary to the popular belief of sensuality 'drying up' as we age, she was the most sensual she's ever felt in her life, but that it hadn't always been this way. I asked her what she thought contributed to this and what had changed. She put it down to one thing: getting to know her cycle. Even though she no longer menstruated, she mapped her cycle to the moon and told me she wished she had this information earlier in life. She recognized in retrospect that at the same time each month, she felt rage-like sensations; sometimes she thought of divorcing her husband, and other times, she wanted to do nothing but make love to him. She now knew that this was a part of her sensual cycle.

The ancient Kama Sutra, whose history we'll explore in more detail in Chapter 11 when we get to the topic of desire, states that different phases of the moon cycle evoke different erogenous zones in the body, which shift through the month. Another ancient text called the *Chandrakalas* informs the arts of sensuality according to the changing phases of the moon; each day has its own sensual spot, with 30 erogenous zones for every day of the month (15 on the left side of the body and 15 on the right). The text was written for any gender to explore for themselves. Indian sexuality educator Seema Anand writes:

> *Starting on the new moon, with the big toe of the left foot for*
> *women and the right foot for men, sexual excitement moves*

up the body for the 15 days of the waxing half of the month until it reaches the head during the full moon and then starts back down again on the opposite side of the body for the next 15 nights (of the waning half) until it reaches the other foot once again.[2]

Below is a description of the erogenous zones on each side of the body, which we can explore throughout the month, according to the phases of the moon. These are meant to be done with a lover, but can be explored on one's own, as well. Progress down one side of the body on days 1–15, then reverse the steps to move back up the body on days 16–30.

▼ **Full Moon, Day 1:** Massage head and hair, or twist around fingers and pull.

▼ **Day 2:** Stroke or kiss the eyes (left first for woman, right first for man).

▼ **Day 3:** Stroke or kiss and bite the lips.

▼ **Day 4:** Stroke or kiss and softly bite the cheeks.

▼ **Day 5:** Rest from a lover and self-pleasure.

▼ **Day 6:** Stroke and scratch the throat.

▼ **Day 7:** Gently touch and scratch the side of the waist.

▼ **Day 8:** Play with the nipples.

▼ **Day 9:** Press, pat, fondle, squeeze, or kiss the whole chest, breasts, nipples, cleavage, and under the breasts.

▼ **Day 10:** Stroke the navel in circles or tap with an open palm.

▼ **Day 11:** Knead, squeeze, and press the buttocks.

- ▼ **Day 12:** Press your lover's knees with your own.

- ▼ **Day 13:** Massage calves and ankles – biting, scratching, kissing, and pressing with your own calves and ankles.

- ▼ **Day 14:** Massage feet or press with your own.

- ▼ **New Moon, Day 15:** Stroke big toe and thumb.

- ▼ **Days 16–30:** Reverse the steps, going up the other side of the body.

The incredible detail with which ancient texts provide sensual guidance is to be celebrated and remembered in our own sensual journey. You can use these steps to enhance your own sensuality and *shakti* through the month. As with any form of arousal, it dies with too much repetition and familiarity. You don't need to follow it day for day, every month. You might use it as a guide for yourself or set a date with a partner to share special time, focusing on the area in alignment with the moon cycle to diversify your connection and spend time on each other in ways you may not otherwise.

We'll now go on to discover another relic that shows us the way the ancient world valued sensuality, which we can all still visit in India.

Goddess Kamakhya

There is a special temple in Guwahati, Assam, India where Goddess Kamakhya is honored. This site is considered the womb of Shakti; the temple has no figure of a goddess deity, but instead, a cave with a natural stone formation that resembles a *yoni*.

The *yoni* represents the sacred space of the vulva, womb, and reproductive organs, and is often depicted as a downward-pointing triangle, symbolizing the sacred source of all manifest creativity and creation. The temple's *yoni* is wet by a natural spring through the year, and devotees go to collect the holy water of this spring, which they either drink for healing purposes or collect in a cloth for good luck.

Miraculously, the spring turns red four days every year, around June 21–25. This is said to be Kamakhya's and the Earth's annual menstrual period. As she bleeds, it's a cause for celebration that attracts thousands of visitors to pass through the temple. Her period invokes a four-day time of rest for the entire community, which is honored in a festival called Ambubachi. Tantric *sadhaks* (spiritual devotees) camp out and concentrate their spiritual practices during this auspicious time.

The temple stems from a myth about the inseparable lovers, Shiva and Shakti. In this myth, Shakti goes by the name Sati. Sati and Shiva are madly in love, but her father, Daksha, doesn't approve of her marrying a matted-haired yogi ascetic and leaving her wealthy life to live with him in the Himalayas. To regain his respect from the community, Daksha hosts a huge party and invites everyone but Shiva. This hurts Sati, who arrives angrily at the party, demanding a reason. Instead, her father shuns her. Her rage and pain consume her, and she jumps into the sacrificial fire. Shiva awakens from his meditation and knows something is wrong. By the time he gets to the party, Sati is dead.

Shiva is inconsolable and takes Sati's remains from the cinders of the sacrificial fire. He carries his lover over his shoulder as he wanders the universe. Eventually, he bumps into Vishnu, the god of preservation, and shares his story. Vishnu has an idea: They will take the remains of Sati's body and spread it across the lands. Each site where one of the goddess's body parts lands will become one of sacred power, known as a *shakti pitha*, where goddess devotees may worship and remember her power until the end of time.

Shiva agrees, and 52 *shakti pithas* are laid across India. Today, we can still visit these sacred sites. Sati's *yoni* is said to have fallen at the site in Assam. This site was discovered by the god of erotic desire, Kama, who was seeking to redeem himself from a punishment from the creator god, Brahma. He paid deep reverence, respect, and devotion to the site of Sati's *yoni*, and the site became a temple known as Kamakhya, meaning 'the one who is revered by Kama.'

The Seasons of Sensuality

There is a certain power in surrendering to the uncontrollable. All that we cannot control reminds us that we are a part of something bigger than ourselves. In recognizing this, we dissolve disconnection and become aligned with our sensual nature. When we become aligned with nature, we are as vast as the night sky and as deep as the ocean. We recognize within ourselves that same higher power. And just as the moon moves the waters, its cycle takes our water-based bodies on its own course through the month, moving our emotional tides and connection to our sensuality. In this way, we don't lose control — we gain alignment.

Where we might put ourselves down for not always feeling sensual or wondering where our sensuality went, I hope this information is a healing balm that can empower you to get to know your inner rhythms and find yourself in peace, wherever you may be in your sensual cycle.

Remember, our sensuality is not only our capacity to feel more pleasure, but to connect to ourselves entirely, in the most intimate of ways. Empowering ourselves with this cyclical wisdom means that we plant our seeds of intention at the right time; know our body's inner rhythms; and honor our body's needs with less self-blame, judgment, and criticism.

There are certain times in our cycle when we might feel more sensual and social, and others when we won't. In some of our seasons, it is better to start off on a new venture or to recoil inward. In some phases, we're more creative, while during others, we allocate time to undertake heavier physical and mental tasks. Seasons exist in nature and inside us, too.

While many menstrual educators in the West map the menstrual cycle according to the four seasons, Ayurveda recognizes six seasons. Therefore, I have mapped the inner sensual cycles to these six seasons, to offer support to the stages where we cross from one phase into another. As you pass through each inner season and phase of the lunar cycle through the month, whether by looking up at the moon or counting the days of your menstrual cycle, notice your energy levels and emotions, how you interact with people and the world around you, what tasks you feel like doing and not doing – and, of course, how sensual you feel.

These seasons are:

▼ *Sisira* – winter

▼ *Vasanta* – spring

▼ *Grisma* – summer

▼ *Varsa* – monsoon

▼ *Sarada* – autumn

▼ *Hemanta* – late autumn

▼ Activity ▼

Tracking Your Sensual Moon Cycle

On the SOSA website (*see p.xxi*) you'll find a Sensual cycle tracker you can download or copy to note what happens at each stage of your cycle. While I share what *could* generally happen, know that these are examples and there's nothing 'wrong' if it doesn't happen in this order for you.

I've added moon indicators so that both people who menstruate and people who don't menstruate can make use of the tracking. Your inner winter and menstruation don't need to align with the new moon, and your inner summer doesn't need to align with the full moon. Cycles also range in days and might be 28 days with ovulation at day 14, as shared on the following pages, or a different duration; it's all unique to you.

Whatever it is, whenever it is, it doesn't matter. What's more important is the process of getting to know your personal sensual cycle and how it feels to you as you attune to your sensations and emotions each day with intimacy and honesty – all while asking yourself what you and your body need. This will inform how you can best look after your unique needs, connect to your sensuality, and nourish your body for optimal balance. For example, on a day when you feel stressed or anxious, firm, grounding touch might be more appealing to the body; on a day when you feel lethargic or numb, light feather tickles might be more enlivening!

As you do this, each month you may start to notice patterns and become more subtly attuned to the sensations, what they mean, and what they're asking for through the month to feel balanced. This will inform what tasks you do according to your energy levels; what kind of social and alone time you plan; what kind of movement supports your phase; and what kind of sensual self-care, intimacy, or interaction would suit you best. Sensuality becomes boring when we use the same patterns over and over again on a body that changes through your cycle. You can use the tracker, an app, or your own journal to expand your sensuality through the month.

Sisira – winter

Days 1–5 of your cycle, first day of menstruation, or the day of the new moon

During this time, the body is focused on its downward flow or releasing the lining of the uterus and the egg. Levels of estrogen and progesterone are at their lowest. The skies are dark. Before the advent of electricity, work would come to a halt as blackness enveloped the skies. This is a time when we are gifted with heightened intuition and access to the experiences and emotions we might otherwise press down. Sexual intercourse is not recommended during this time, due to the downward *vayu*, but soft, sensual self-care can be very nourishing. Offer yourself restorative practices and avoid inversions; nourish your body with healthy foods, lots of rest, journaling, reflection, and self-care.

Vasanta – spring

Days 5–9, beginning of follicular phase, or waxing crescent to first quarter moon

A new egg is being prepared to release; a sliver of the moon is illuminated. This is a time of renewed energy and a good period for planting seeds for new projects and intentions. The moon is starting to grow. With the increase in energy, your mood and emotions may provide support for personal development. You may want to change your sheets, make home improvements, and enjoy sexual pleasure during this season, as energy returns to the body. You may also want to engage in new activities, make investments, or undertake more dynamic *asana* or physical exercise in this time.

Grisma – summer

Days 10–14, follicular phase to ovulation, or waxing gibbous to full moon

These are the days running up to ovulation when your body is preparing an egg to release from an ovary. This is also your most fertile phase. The temperature of the body rises due to the increase in progesterone and *agni*, the fire element that is activated in the body. The moon is becoming more full, and the sky is bright. Use this illumination to explore and build connections with people and projects. Energy is focused outward, so it's a good time for public speaking, sales, or workshops. You may feel extra adventurous in your sensuality; you could explore new kinks, outfits, toys, or activities with yourself or your partner. Be careful not to overdo this period, as you may experience burnout in the next.

Varsa – monsoon

Days 14–18, ovulation to luteal phase, or full moon to waning gibbous

The egg travels down the fallopian tube toward the uterus. The full moon starts to wane. This period leads to an increase of focus, so use this time to undertake administrative tasks you might not have the energy or time for in other periods. You may want to declutter your inbox, clean your home and wardrobe, get nitty and gritty with your spreadsheets, and crunch your numbers. You may also want to engage in sensual acts for hydrating the body: drinking plenty of water, enjoying a spa, or getting oil massages, or *abhyanga*, to hydrate the skin. Your yoga practice might look more fluid and flowing.

Sarada – autumn

Days 18–22, luteal/secretory phase, or waning gibbous to last quarter

The lining of the uterus thickens in preparation for potential pregnancy. The moon is in its third or last quarter, and there's a shift from outward to inward. If you've got unfinished projects at work or around the home, it's time to complete them. Use this time to reflect on what is no longer serving you emotionally. If there's anything you've been holding in your heart that's been left unsaid, it's a good time to have the conversation. Physically, you may want to use this time to engage in releasing, shaking, and activities that give you a sense of catharsis. Your self-care activities may include lymphatic massage, exfoliation, or dry brushing. Sensually, you'll have more clarity and could use this time to discuss your desires and engage in slower self-pleasure and sex.

Hemanta – late autumn

Days 22–28, luteal/secretory phase to menstruation, or last quarter to waning crescent

If pregnancy does not occur, the uterus prepares to release the egg and lining, so you might experience discomfort, bloating, or changes in your skin, body, and mood as your hormones change to prepare for the expulsion of physical and emotional toxins. The last sliver of the moon remains. Make use of your hormonal shifts to go more deeply into your creative endeavors. Physically, you may want to move into more restorative balancing practices. Engage in creative activities like journaling, painting, or any projects to channel your inner expression and fluctuations. Sensual indulgence and sex can be particularly enjoyable!

Integration

1. What is your relationship with your menstrual/sensual moon cycle?

2. What did you learn about the menstrual cycle growing up (even if you don't menstruate)?

3. What are the erogenous zones that activate *shakti* or sensuality in your body?

4. What season are you currently in? How do you feel?

KEY TAKEAWAYS

~ Sensuality can be explored through the ancient science of life, Ayurveda, which puts us in sync with our inner and outer seasons.

~ According to Ayurveda, the three *doshas* (known as *vata*, *pitta*, and *kapha*) rule nature and the functioning of the body, and can be referred to in order to empower a sense of inner balance.

~ The *vayus*, or winds, determine the flow of energy through the body and also rule the menstrual cycle, as well as its gifts of intuition and rest.

~ Ancient Tantric texts mapped the sensual erogenous zones to the phases of the moon, and we can use their wisdom to playfully explore our own sensuality, especially as arousal waxes and wanes throughout the month.

~ In ancient India, menstruation was a sacred function, and the myth of Shakti's *yoni* is well and alive in the temple of Goddess Kamakhya in Assam – where the water still flows red four days of the year, miraculously paying homage to the *shakti* of this sacred place.

~ The seasons of our sensuality can be mapped to match the six seasons that were acknowledged in the sister sciences of Ayurveda, Tantra, and Yoga (and can also be mapped to match our menstrual cycle, as well as the moon cycle). With this awareness, we can track our sensuality and what we might need to understand ourselves more intimately.

CHAPTER 4

Knowing Your Sensual Rivermap (Yoga)

Through centuries of self-inquiry and study, the ancestors of Tantra gave us a gift to access deeper sensuality and to open a network to know our source and spirit. I like to call this network the Tantric Roadmap or Sensual Rivermap. In this chapter, we will get to know this map, from its source point to its coordinates in the body, where we can harness sensual energy and direct it for healing, rejuvenation, vitality, pleasure, creativity, and expansion.

A Mystical Convergence

As my enthusiasm for working in the legal system started to fade, I began to luxuriate in my lunch break — counting the hours until it came and stretching out every minute possible. I'd go to the same restaurant every day; it had quick service and a good choice of carbs to tide me over while I sat thinking over my options.

One day, it was so busy in there, the waiter asked if I would be willing to share my two-seater table with another solo diner. I didn't see why not and continued to pour my attention into the pages of my book. The other diner, a 40-something-year-old Chinese woman, sat down and pulled out a book. There was a familiar and mutual silence between us, which I appreciated. As the waiter came over, I ordered in English and she ordered in Mandarin. The waiter laughed, as we had ordered the same starter, main, and drink. I looked up and caught the name of her book: *The Bhagavad Gita*.

The first thought was that the order was a cute coincidence between two diners on an idle lunchtime in the world's most populated and busy city. The second sign, the book she was reading, made me break the comfortable silence with a gentle 'Radhe, Radhe.' This is a Sanskrit greeting to honor Shakti and Radha, the counterpart of the well-known blue-skinned Krishna (an *avatar* of the god of preservation, Vishnu).

The woman looked up from her pages and smiled. 'You know this text?' I smiled back and shared the story of how my father was a monk in the Hare Krishna movement through the eighties; he'd helped set up the temple in Paris and later ran a temple art café in the premier arrondissement of the city, selling beautiful sculptures and artifacts by day and sharing delicious vegetarian food by night. We shared our love and thoughts about the teachings of Krishna riding in his chariot — a symbol of the mind, the soul, and the vehicle of life.

Every few weeks or so, I would cross paths with this mystical woman, and each time, I experienced a beautiful unveiling of source and spirit. This was the kind of encounter you didn't have to make an appointment for, yet she almost always appeared at the perfect time to deliver a poignant message.

During one lunch break, she walked into the restaurant and came to sit opposite me. This time, she shared that she was writing a book about the spirituality of money. In China, businesses, homes, and establishments will often greet you with the sound of running water out the front. The flow of water trickling down a fountain represents prosperity, abundance, and motion. Our conversation spiraled to the running waters of the world, and she mentioned that during her latest holiday, she took her family to a specific point halfway across the island, where the sea meets a river.

In geographical terms, the place where fresh water meets coastal water is known as an estuary, and holds potential for hydrokinetic energy production. At this conjunction point, where two currents of water meet, a strong energy emerges to clear blocks, traumas, and impurities resting in the body and soul, and replenishes it with abundant life force, much like our own enriching encounters. I asked how she felt after her dip and her smile said it all. 'Just try it,' she replied. That was the last time I saw her.

Your Sacred Sensual Rivers

There are seven major holy rivers running through India: Ganga, Yamuna, Indus, Saraswati, Godarvi, Narmada, and Kaveri. Each one is considered a manifestation of Shakti, a goddess who is to be honored, loved, and respected for how she nourishes the lands.

The Haridwar River is the meeting place of the Ganga, Saraswati, and Yamuna rivers. *Hare* (another name for Shiva or God) and *dwar* (which literally means 'door') makes it a doorway to God for thousands of pilgrims who bathe at the confluence of the three rivers, known as *Triveni Sangam*, every year. The space is considered a liminal portal, halfway between the spiritual and material realms. Here, ashes are often scattered to carry the soul to meet spirit.

As on the lands of India, there are rivers that run through the body. These are known as *nadis* — and like the rivers that carry water and the veins that carry blood, *nadis* carry the currents of energy that flow through each being.

In Western medicine, if someone presents with a sexual dysfunction, such as vaginismus or erectile dysfunction, what is physically visible and quantifiable is studied. For example, the muscles of the vagina involuntarily contract or spasm at the prospect of penetration, or there is not enough blood reaching the penis to sustain an erection. Medicine, Viagra, and numbing cream to treat the physical manifestation are given.

In Eastern medicine systems, it is recognized that in order for our minds and bodies (including our sexual organs) to function, we must consider two essential components: the gross form and the subtle form. The gross form is the material body — our flesh, tissues, bones, hair, blood, excrements — and the subtle form is the energetic channels composed of the *nadis*, of which there are around 72,000 in the body. These *nadis* serve as a blueprint for our physical cells to organize themselves.

Many daily practices in the East cultivate this flow of energy that represents life force. In India, it's called *prana*; in Japan, it's called *ki*; and in China, it's called *qi*. Highly skilled martial arts such as kung fu and tai chi are practices that cultivate deep concentration one's *qi*. All of us could stand to learn about the network of *prana* within the body, as it is an innate intelligence that maintains homeostasis.

Having seen the power of this flow of energy when I witnessed a young boy, no older than 10, chop a block of wood with his hand in the Shaolin temple of China, I become more curious about cultivating life-force energy. We can harvest energy from air, food, and water, as well as particular practices that cultivate and store energy in the body. In Tantra and Yoga, just like the conjunction of water currents that meet to create a high density of energy, the body hosts a network of centers where the rivers of energy intersect. These energy centers are known as *chakras.*

Your Sensual Rivermap

Much like the pilgrims visiting the transition points across the holy rivers in India to offer their devotion, we can also make pilgrimage to the *chakra* points of the body — to receive wisdom, expand our sensation, and unblock the obstacles that are laid around them through our experiences.

Working with our chakras *helps us in the most practical way to become more fully embodied, sensual beings.*

In his foundational book on the *chakras, Laya Yoga,* Shyam Sundar Goswami brings together knowledge from the *Upanishads,* the *Tantras,* and the Puranas, ancient texts that reveal the powers of these sacred energy centers. He translates *chakra* to the 'wheel of a carriage,' 'a potter's wheel,' and 'a circular weapon.'[1]

Each wheel is a vortex of vital life-force energy that circles in particular areas of the body. Due to *The Serpent Power,* a book by Sir John Woodroffe that was written about a hundred years ago, most of us in the West are taught that there are only seven *chakras,* which are considered to be particularly large reservoirs of energy. But in traditional Tantric systems, just as many streams come together to form a great river, these seven *chakras* are supported by energy carried through the *nadis* from the others, which are usually found a few inches away.

According to ancient traditions, there are up to 114 *chakras* in the body, made up of primary, secondary, and micro *chakras* connected through the network of 72,000 *nadis* carrying energy through their channels between the *chakras*. A *chakra* is essentially any intersectional energy point. You can get to know this incredible network for your own physical, mental, emotional, energetic, sexual, sensual, and spiritual health.

Some lesser-known but important *chakras* to note are found in each ear, above each breast/chest, at the intersection of the clavicle, in each palm, in the soles of your feet, above each eye, in the reproductive organs, in the liver, in the stomach, in the spleen, in the back of each knee, underneath your heart, and behind your solar plexus, to name a few!

The *chakras* may have been misused in popular culture or questioned because they belong to the subtle rather than gross material body; however, they run along the spine and map to the endocrine and nervous system, often meeting at the confluence of nerve bundles and glands. As Neale Donald Walsch reminds us in his book, *Conversations with God*:

> *Emotion is energy in motion. When you move energy, you create effect. If you move enough energy, you create matter. Matter is energy conglomerated. Moved around. Shoved together. If you manipulate energy long enough in a certain way, you get matter. Every Master understands this law. It is the alchemy of the universe. It is the secret of all life.*[2]

Our emotions are energy in motion, so inevitably, the emotions we feel through the experiences we have had over the course of our lives affect the flow of *nadis* and *chakras*. Our subtle body forms a blueprint for our material body, and if energy blockages are left untreated, they will manifest in the physical form, creating holding patterns in our musculature[3] and organs, so one of the best ways we can look after ourselves is by looking after our energy flow.

As neuroscience now confirms, 'the body keeps the score.' The *chakras* are often where experiences get stored, affecting the function of our cells, tissues, and organs. When we experience trauma, as we will explore in Chapter 6, it can get stored in the cell memory, blocking our energetic rivers and reservoirs and cutting off an essential supply of nourishment to our bodies. Where our inner rivers run dry of energy, we may experience pain, discomfort, dis-ease, infection, or numbness in particular areas. Where the rivers are flowing, we experience healthy functioning and flow of all our internal systems, as well as deeper connection to our sensations and sensuality.

There is a Chinese proverb that states, 'Flowing water never stagnates,' so our Sensual Rivermap indicates to us where to unlock and unblock our sensual energy.

> *Our* chakras *don't only show us what's wrong; they show us where we are strong, where we have come from, what we have experienced, what we like, and who we are. They empower us with a tool to explore where to evolve next.*

Let's meander to the *chakras* and the pathways that connect them, with practices to explore, unblock, and expand sensual energy.

Getting to Know Your Sensual Rivermap

Of the 72,000 *nadis* carrying the currents of energy around the body, there are 14 important ones. Of those 14, there are three you need to know: *ida*, *pingala*, and *sushumna*.

Ida nadi is the channel on the left side of the body, and *pingala nadi* is the channel on the right side.

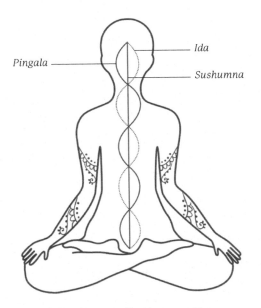

Pingala

Ida

Sushumna

Ida, pingala, and *sushumna* nadis

Ida nadi is the receptive side, ruled by the moon and associated with Shakti; *pingala nadi* holds active sun energy and is associated with Shiva. On either side of the spine are two holes that are like pipes for all the nerves to pass through; *ida* and *pingala* move through this passage. The currents of *ida* and *pingala* cross, like the great rivers. They form the shape of a DNA helix (found in Tantra long before the scientific discovery of DNA in 1953) between the major *chakras* and join at the sixth *chakra* in the center of the head, representing union or nonduality.

Between the two *nadis*, running along the spine, is the central channel of the body, the *sushumna nadi*, containing the *brahma nadi*, which opens the higher channel of the subtle body. *Sushumna* is very fine, begins in the root of the spine, and goes all the way up to the crown. The network of *nadis* and *chakras* are connected with this central *sushumna nadi*. Inside the *sushumna* is a *nadi* named *vajra*, and inside that is an even subtler *nadi* called *chitrini*, through which *kundalini shakti* passes.[4]

When *kundalini shakti* is roused in the root of the body, it passes through the waters of the sensual center, *Svadhistana*, where it transforms into waves that move through the body. Sexual energy then transforms from a sneeze in the pelvis outward, into currents facing inward that can move around the body to clear blocks, nourish cells, and create a deeper connection to our sensations. This inward drawing of sexual energy and transformation into sensual waves helps us make space for energy that nourishes the entire body, mind, and spirit.

One must act with caution when working with *kundalini shakti* and go slowly and consistently through the pathways to establish grounding, familiarity, safety, and practice, all with the right guidance. If *kundalini shakti* moves too fast up the *sushumna nadi*, which can be the case with intense practices done without the right supervision, the energy can be unleashed too quickly and cause a lot of damage in the body and mind — something that's known as *kundalini psychosis*.

Therefore, if you have a history of any familial or personal mental illnesses or personality disorders, you should not undertake any of the practices on the following pages without working specifically with medical consent. Tantra Yoga is a way to experience *kundalini* with consciousness and awareness of how to transform it, rather than shoot it up with intensity. If we are looking to go straight from root to crown for out-of-body experiences that take us into different realms, even spiritual practice can be a form of escapism or an addiction with a drug-like quality. I offer a gentle invitation with love and care for where you take this information with you on your personal spiritual, sensual, or Tantric path.

The Seven Major Watermills

Energy can be sourced in a multiplicity of ways, and there is an immeasurable and infinite amount of energy available to us. On the following pages, I outline the different ways you can source energy to heal, nourish, balance, and expand the seven major *chakras* in the body. You'll find their location; the affected gland, organ, and areas of the body; the element of nature that can balance them; the sense associated with the area; the *bija mantra* that can be chanted (we'll explore this more deeply in Chapter 10); the color that can be worn; the foods that can be eaten; activities and balancing practices that help to cultivate energy in that area; and the visual representation of the *chakra*, which forms a lotus with different numbers of petals as you move up the spine.

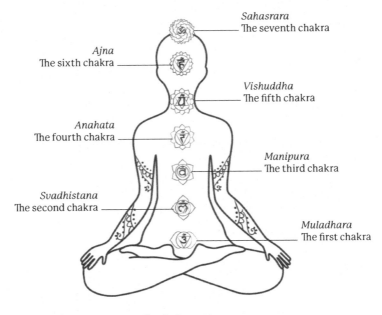

Sahasrara
The seventh chakra

Ajna
The sixth chakra

Vishuddha
The fifth chakra

Anahata
The fourth chakra

Manipura
The third chakra

Svadhistana
The second chakra

Muladhara
The first chakra

The chakra system

If you'd like to learn more about the *asana* (posture) practices in this chapter, I encourage you to join SOSA's online Tantra Yoga community or Pleasure Pathways Course (*see p.xxi*). In addition, Swami Satyananda Saraswati's book, *Asana Pranayama Mudra Bandha*, is a wonderful resource.

First Chakra

Name: *Mulhadhara*; *mulha* meaning the 'root of existence'

Location: between anus and genitals, the perineal region

Affecting: adrenal gland, kidneys, feet, legs, pelvis, hips

Element: earth

Sense: smell

Mantra: *lam*

Color: red

Lotus: four petals

In balance: grounded, stable, sure, safe, connected, able, anchored, rooted, trusting

Out of balance: fearful, traumatized, disconnected, sluggish, lethargic, greedy, materialistic, financially insecure, moves homes a lot, is resistant to change

What to Know

We are opening the red doors to our body's Sensual Rivermap. As we move into the root, we encounter the first watermill, which create a foundation for our energy practices. This is the physical and energetic seat of *kundalini shakti*, the sexual energy represented in Tantric practices as a serpent coiled at the base of the spine and pelvic bowl.

This is the most important *chakra* in our sensual exploration, as it forms the basis of feeling safe physically, emotionally, energetically, and spiritually. Before we explore our sensuality, we need to ensure we feel safe to do so in our bodies. Otherwise, contractions from our tension, trauma, and stress held in this area will keep our sexual energy pushed down and suppressed.

The first *chakra* is concerned with your survival instincts. The practices to bring balance to this area invite you to ground into the earth; to ensure you feel secure in your physical, mental, financial, energetic, and emotional body; and to become more familiar with your pelvic bowl and the *kundalini shakti* energy.

Balancing Practices

Yoga: *mulha bandha* (root lock), *ashwini mudra* (anus gesture), *vrksasana* (tree pose), *malasana* (garland pose), *utkata konasana* (goddess pose), *badokonasana* (bound angle pose/butterfly pose), *tadasana* (mountain pose), *sukhasana* (easy pose), *padmasana* (lotus pose), *balasana* (child's pose), *savasana* (corpse pose)

Pranayama: *nadi shodhana* (alternate nostril breathing)

Activities: body scan, foot massage, looking after home, reviewing financial security, therapy for unprocessed trauma, weight lifting, climbing, trampolining, jumping, skipping, twerking, *garba* dance, aromatherapy, using different essential oils on your pulse points, incense

Sensuality: grounding touch, sharing worries/intentions/desires, affirmations, hugging

Relationships: connecting with relationships from childhood, family, friends

Foods: vegetables grown under the earth, kidney beans, paprika, cloves, red meat, tofu, red fruits and vegetables

Nature: walking barefoot on earth, grass, sand; exploring forests

Journal questions: *Do I have enough for my basic survival? What do I fear? Who can I trust? How was my childhood? What is/was my relationship with my parents? What is my relationship with money? What do I need to feel safe? What do I need to feel secure? Have I experienced trauma? What is toxic for me? What am I letting go of?*

Affirmations: *I am safe now. I am secure, grounded, centered, strong, rooted, and trusting.*

Second Chakra

Name: *Svadhistana; svad* meaning 'taste' or 'pleasure'; the dwelling place of the self

Location: three to four fingers below the navel

Affecting: sexual organs, ovaries, testicles, prostate, vulva, penis, bladder, kidney, lower intestine, lower back, lower abdomen, sacrum, pelvis, hips

Element: water

Sense: taste

Mantra: *vam*

Color: vermilion orange

Lotus: six petals

In balance: emotional security, pleasure, sensuality, flow, creativity, play, passion, ease, sexual fulfillment

Out of balance: depression, numbness, addiction, menstrual disorders, sexual dysfunction, fertility issues, urinary issues, creative blocks, lower back pain, kidney stones, difficulty adapting to change, shame, guilt, rigidity, dry skin, stiffness

What to Know

Next, as we flow through the Sensual Rivermap, we move into the orange dwelling place of sensuality. This second watermill is known as *Svadhistana*, where sexual energy is transformed into sensual energy and *prana*. This sensual *shakti* energy communicates to us through the sensations that carry sacred messages to us through the day and night. It invites us to pay attention to these sensations, which form the currents of emotion that drive our desires and actions.

The second *chakra* can be constricted by sexual trauma, fear of intimacy, and disconnection or suppression of our emotions. This seat is not just about reproduction or sex — it is also the source of our creative power.

Balancing Practices

Yoga: *bitilasana marjaryasana* (cat cow), *bhujangasana* (cobra pose), *vyaghrasana dandayamana bharmanasana* (knee-to-nose vinyasa), *pada hastasana* (standing forward bend with hands under feet), *paschimottanasana* (seated forward bend), *chandra namaskar* (moon salutations), *yoni mudra* (womb gesture), *uddhiyana bandha* (flying upward lock)

Pranayama: *ujjayi* breath (breathing with a soft ocean sound)

Activities: working with the pubococcygeus (PC) muscle, drinking lots of water, belly dancing, partner dances (such as salsa, bachata, kizomba, zouk, etc.), skating, hula hooping, oil massage (*abhyanga*), cooking, self-pleasure, sex, making art, connecting to creativity, decorating the home, water sports

Sensuality: savoring the taste of your food, focusing on foreplay, oil/fluid touch

Relationships: nurturing sexual intimacy, pleasure, playfulness in relationships

Foods: juicy fruits, watery legumes, soups, orange foods, red lentils, sweet potatoes, fish, oranges, carrots, peaches, papayas, cucumbers, butterfly pea tea

Nature: swimming; going to the beach; visiting rivers, waterfalls, lakes

Journal questions: *What sensations and emotions do I feel in this moment? What are my favorite creative activities? What brings me pleasure? What are my favorite flavors? What are my favorite intimate experiences? What are uncomfortable intimate experiences I've had? Have I experienced any sexual trauma? What am I passionate about? Have I been able to express my emotions freely through my life?*

Affirmations: *I am sensual, sexual, flowing, creative, juicy, and passionate. I deserve to feel the full spectrum of my emotions. I deserve to feel pleasure.*

Third Chakra

Name: *Manipura*; *mani* meaning 'shining gem,' *pura* meaning 'city'; the city of jewels

Location: a few fingers above the navel, between the ribs

Affecting: solar plexus, colon, spleen, stomach, liver, pancreas, stomach, mid-spine

Element: fire

Sense: sight

Mantra: *ram*

Color: yellow

Lotus: 10 petals

In balance: self-worth, empowerment, courage, motivation, energy, purpose, willpower, assertiveness, discipline, clarity, nourishment, healthy digestion of emotions and food

Out of balance: anger, anxiety, frustration, self-righteousness, unrealistic expectations, slow digestive function, tendency to overeat, low self-esteem, control issues, digestive disorders, diabetes, eating disorders, allergies, difficulty setting boundaries

What to Know

As we sail through our Sensual Rivermap, we encounter the third watermill and ignite our yellow inner spark in the solar plexus, known as *Manipura*. This is located between the ribs and is a network that connects and communicates with all our organs.

Working with this area fuels a fire to feed our inner confidence and courage. This fire seeks to illuminate our self-worth and sensual power while keeping material illusion and ego at bay. Too little fuel and the fire burns out; too much fuel and the fire could be wild and dangerous for us and others.

In sensuality, the third *chakra* represents power play and how intimate we allow ourselves to be with others. Intimacy requires vulnerability. Nourishment comes through both food and connection. Tantra gives us tools to empower ourselves with the ability to keep our inner fire burning at the perfect temperature, so it can fuel our growth, nourishment, and expansion while keeping us warm and safe.

Meet this fuel at the center of your body and let its flames burn a pathway into your sovereign sensual power.

Balancing Practices

Yoga: *surya namaskar* (sun salutations), *dhanurasana* (bow pose), *ardha matsyendrasana* (half spinal twist), *kumbakasana* (plank pose), *malasana* (garland pose), *vajrasana* (thunderbolt pose) *purottanasana* (upward plank pose), *virabhadrasana* (warrior pose), *parvritta trikonasana* (revolved triangle pose), *utkatasana* (chair pose), *vajroli mudra* (lightning *mudra*)

Pranayama: *kapalabhati* (breath of fire), *trataka* (candle gazing)

Activities: stomach massage, taking photos or videos, aerobic exercise, running, sunbathing, wearing jewelry, shaking, boxing, screaming, setting boundaries

Sensuality: admiring yourself, eye gazing with a lover, activating touch, candlelit evenings, exploring boundaries/power play

Relationships: nurturing connections in your work or professional field

Foods: bananas, pineapples, lemons, wheat, yellow split peas, ginger, turmeric, squash, whole grains, brown rice, quinoa, millet, bulgur

Nature: building, sitting around or cooking over a fire, watching sunset and sunrise

Journal questions: *What are my ambitions, goals, and dreams? What is something I'm seeking courage to do? What was one of my most courageous moments? What drives me? What emotional experiences am I still digesting? What foods feel easy/not easy to digest? What do I feel angry about? I am worthy because...*

Affirmations: *I am courageous, confident, empowered, motivated, ambitious, capable, and worthy.*

Fourth Chakra

Name: *Anahata*, meaning 'unhurt, unstruck, unbeaten'

Location: center of chest

Affecting: arms, hands, shoulders, chest, breasts, ribs, upper back, thorax, lungs, heart, thymus

Element: air

Sense: sight

Mantra: *yam*

Color: green

Lotus: 12 petals

In balance: love, nonjudgment, empathy, kindness, open heart, forgiveness, self-care, harmony, unconditional love, compassion, transformation

Out of balance: loneliness, criticism of self and others, jealousy, narcissism, asthma, allergies, grief, abandonment, heart and lung problems, poor circulation, shyness, social anxiety, suspicion, codependency, isolation, clinginess

What to Know

Next, we sail into the fourth watermill — a green temple of transformation, where we open the doors to the most intimate of spaces in our heart and lungs. This center invites each breath as a loving caress of our inner world with an invitation not to seek for love, but as Rumi says, to melt the barriers we have built against it.

As we lay the grief, heartbreak, regrets, disappointments, and armor we have built to rest, we emerge into a space where we can wear our scars with strength and enter a deeper connection with ourselves and the world around us. The heart is another gate through which we can access our sexual energy to transform into sensual energy or *prana*. Whatever we bring into *Anahata* has the capacity to transform, transmute, and expand.

Balancing Practices

Yoga: *setu bandha savangasana* (bridge pose), *salamba bhujangasana* (sphinx pose), *natrajasana* (dancer's pose), *garudasana* (eagle pose), *chakrasana* (wheel pose), *utrasana* (camel pose), *camatkarasana* (wild thing), *hridaya mudra* (spiritual heart gesture), chin *mudra* (hand seal/gesture to redirect energy)

Pranayama: *dirga pranayama* (three-part breath)

Activities: gratitude list, *metta* (loving kindness) meditation, breathwork, acts of self-care, caring for hands, opening windows at home for fresh air, breast massage, ribcage clearance, shoulder and upper-back massage, badminton, tennis, cricket, netball, basketball, *Ho'oponopono* (forgiveness and letting go) meditation

Sensuality: expressing love to yourself and another, feather-light touch

Relationships: nurturing connection with people you love

Foods: leafy greens, broccoli, pot herbs, spinach, kale, green tea, avocados, celery, salad leaves, limes, bok choy, apples

Nature: visiting mountains, countryside, and grasslands

Journal questions: *What am I grieving? Is there anything I have not forgiven? Where in my life have I been disappointed/hurt? Are there any parts of myself or others I hold in judgment? How do I best receive and give love? What is my love language (gifts, quality time, acts of service, physical touch, words of affirmation)? What are the love languages of my loved ones? Three compliments I give myself now are...*

Affirmations: I am love consciousness, compassionate, forgiving and open to both receiving and giving love with abundance

Fifth Chakra

Name: *Vishuddha*, meaning 'pure' or 'purification'
Location: throat

Affecting: thyroid, larynx, voice, neck, throat, jaw, ears, mouth, teeth, gums, upper shoulders

Element: space/ether

Sense: sound

Mantra: *ham*

Color: blue/turquoise

Lotus: 16 petals

In balance: communicating with clarity, speaking one's truth, confidence expressing opinions, good listening, social awareness of others' emotions when speaking

Out of balance: difficulty expressing oneself, overtalking as a defense, shyness, inability to speak confidently, fear expressing opinions, tendency to talk more than listen, fear of embarrassment, habitual lying, overinflation of reality, fear of making noise or letting go, thyroid problems, scratchy voice, sore throat, tonsil problems, bleeding gums, ear problems

What to Know

We sail over to the fifth watermill to meet our own unapologetic expression. As we visit *Vishuddha* in the throat, we open the doors to the instrument of our voice.

This center invites us to dance to the conversation of life, speaking our authentic truth and listening with ears of love. As the center of purification, it offers us a direct path to paint our inner energy in the outer world through sound. It is also about the way we speak to ourselves.

In our bodies, there is a direct connection with the throat and pelvis, anatomically and energetically. Tension held in the jaw and armoring around the throat can appear in the pelvis. Speak your truth and hear your sensual serpent rise to your call. Tune the beat of your heart to the sound of your soul, and welcome home the harmony of your inner orchestra.

Balancing Practices

Yoga: chanting *mantras*, *seturasana* (bridge pose), *matsyasana* (fish pose), *salamba sarvangasana* (supported shoulder stand), *halasana* (plow pose), *sucirandrasana* (threat the needle), *ardha matsyendrasana* (half spinal twist), *jalandhara bandha* (throat lock)

Pranayama: *simhasana* (lion's breath)

Activities: singing, toning, humming, giving compliments, conscious communication techniques such as nonviolent communication, talk therapy, journaling, making art, listening to music, playing music, learning an instrument, creating space for self-care (physical, emotional, mental), decluttering

Sensuality: words of affirmation, whispering compliments, kissing, energetic touch

Relationships: nurturing communication with people who share the same hobbies

Foods: blueberries, honey, lemons, blackberries, lemongrass, elderberry, sage

Nature: looking at the stars, moon, space, and planets; visiting wide open spaces in nature

Journal questions: *What is the ratio of speaking/listening in my daily conversations? What is my favorite mode of communication (verbal/nonverbal/creative)? What modalities can I use to express my feelings (creativity)? If I listen to the script in my head, what does it tell me about the relationship with myself? How do I feel* *expressing my opinion at home, work, relationships, and with other groups in my life? Was my voice valued growing up?* You can also choose to write a letter expressing something you have always wanted to say to someone but never have (it doesn't matter if you send it or not – you can practice expressing).

Affirmations: *I am empowered to speak my truth. I express clearly and openly. My voice matters. I am comfortable with silence. I am authentic. It is safe to show my true self.*

Sixth Chakra

Name: *Ajna*, meaning 'perceive/command'

Location: center of head (not just forehead, but the middle of head/brain)

Affecting: pineal gland, eyes, head, scalp, sinus

Element: light

Sense: sight

Mantra: *om*

Color: indigo

Lotus: two petals

In balance: intuition, imagination, ease falling asleep and resting, manifestation, mystical visions, visionary thoughts, intelligence, good memory, constructive rather than critical attitude

Out of balance: cloudy thoughts, difficulty visualizing, difficulty sleeping, sore/tired eyes, anxious/distracting/harmful thoughts, difficulty connecting to sensations, lack of intuition, avoidance of reality, naive optimism, self-critical or loathing tendencies, headaches

What to Know

We sail into our sixth watermill, where the indigo lights in our sacred temple illuminate a path to be reunited with our inner teacher. As we pay pilgrimage to *Ajna* at the center of the mind's eye, we open ourselves to the intuitive wisdom within.

This center links to the pineal gland, the motherboard that secretes the sleep and reproductive hormones in the body. It invites us to find stillness between the thoughts that separate us from trusting our intuitive nature. Both hemispheres of the brain, in balance, work together to help us move past dualistic thinking.

Where the two eyes see, the third eye senses, with the sensations of the body as its sacred messengers. With a practice of focus, we are offered a source of light to see our own sensual sacredness. As the sensual serpent rises to the mind, she gifts us the lightning power of intuition and manifesting with our minds. When out of balance, we can feel closed to the world and hazy-eyed. When in balance, we experience clarity, foresight, and deep trust in life.

Balancing Practices

Yoga: *trataka* (candle-gazing meditation), *jala neti* (sinus cleansing), *vrksasana* (tree pose), *garudasana* (eagle pose), *padmasana* (lotus pose), *balasana* (child's pose), *makrasana* (crocodile pose), *shalamba sarvangasana* (supported shoulder stand), *dandayamana bharmanasana* (balancing table pose), *ardha chandrasana* (half-moon pose), *adho mukha vrksasana* (handstand), *adho mukha svanasana* (downward-facing dog), *prasarita padottanasana* (wide-legged forward bend), *yoga nidra* (yogic sleep), *shambhavi mudra* (eyebrow-center gazing gesture)

Pranayama: *brahmari* breath (bee breath)

Activities: *netra shakti vikasaka* (eye movement practices), meditating on the breath, sungazing, sunbathing, reading, decorating one's home, visualization, coloring, daydreaming, photography, drawing, Sudoku, word searches, board games, memory games, dream journaling, creating an evening wind-down ritual, writing down one's thoughts with freewriting

Sensuality: eye gazing, blindfolding, sharing thoughts and ideas

Relationships: nurturing intellectual connections and inspiring conversations

Foods: walnuts, almonds and other nuts, seeds, goji berries, grapes

Nature: watching sunrise and sunset

Journal questions: *When was a time I trusted my imagination? Were there times I didn't follow my intuition but wish I had? Do I have recurring dreams at night? What are my dreams for my life, and what do they look like? Do I have intuition about a particular ongoing experience in my life right now? What do I love, what do I hate, and why?*

Affirmations: *I trust myself. I trust my intuition. I trust my inner teacher. I see with clarity.*

Seventh Chakra

Name: *Sahasrara*, meaning 'thousand-petaled'

Location: crown of the head

Affecting: pituitary gland, hypothalamus, brain, nervous system

Element: thought

Sense: spirit/all senses

Mantra: silence

Color: white/violet

Lotus: thousand petals

In balance: sensing oneself as being part of something bigger, connection to higher power, wisdom, sense of community, connection to one's spirit, awareness of both material and subtle energy, ability to see bigger picture, mysticism, transcendental ideas

Out of balance: spiritual bypassing, disconnection, loneliness, confusion, distraction, lack of focus, hyper-spiritualization, lack of connection to material world

Things to Know

Our Sensual Rivermap culminates in the seventh watermill at *Sahasrara*, where we meet our spiritual center, connecting our material and subtle bodies to a higher power. It is not connected to a particular sense but is responsible for integrating all the senses collected from the other *chakras*.

As the bookend, it shares a connection with the root; the crown and root were connected in our embryonic development. When we become aware of this center, it allows us to feel the deep interconnectedness between ourselves, other humans, and the universe. We can receive and share energy with the universe, which has an unlimited supply, but first we need to work through all the *chakras* that stop us from realizing we are part of a bigger picture.

There are less specific practices for the crown, as it is the culmination of all the work to open and flow energy from the previous *chakras*. It reminds us that we are spiritual beings having a human experience, and that when we respond to the call of our sensual spirit, as you are doing with this book, we are saying yes not only to our own evolution but that of all living beings around us.

Balancing Practices

Yoga: *savasana* (corpse pose), *yoga nidra* (yogic sleep), *balasana* (child's pose), *supta badokanasana* (sleeping butterfly pose), *sirsasana* (head stand), *salamba sirsasana* (supported head stand), *salamba sarvangasana* (supported shoulder stand), *padmasana* (lotus pose), *sukhasana* (easy pose), *padma mudra* (thousand-petaled gesture).

Pranayama: Inhale *so*, exhale *ham* (*so ham* means 'I am that,' which constitutes everything: divine reality/truth/universe)

Activities: spiritual practices, meditating, praying, creating an altar, forming a relationship with your higher power, maintaining that relationship consistently with devotional practices, head and scalp massage, bringing sacredness to your life/work/relationships

Sensuality: meditating and sharing spiritual practices together

Relationships: nurturing relationships with people who support your spiritual evolution and allow for philosophical conversations

Foods: fasting, detoxing, water, lavender, sage, frankincense, juniper

Nature: climbing to the peak of a mountain and enjoying the view above and below

Journal questions: *How connected do I feel to my higher power/ the divine/the universe? What helps me foster this connection and communicate with it? Did I have a religious upbringing? How was this experience for me? What does my own relationship with spirit*

look like now? If I connected to my higher power right now, what would it tell me? How can I offer my service as an act of devotion to the world?

Affirmations: I trust my higher power. I am a part of something bigger. I am loved and cared for. I am spirit. I am soul. I am divine. I am connected to spirit. I have purpose.

▼ Activities ▼

The SENSFUL Method

SENSFULness is the new mindfulness! SENSFUL can be applied to all of life: meditating, walking, eating, lovemaking, anything! I created this method so it can be mapped to the *chakra* system and enable us to be more embodied in each moment. We'll use this method as a basis for practices in Part II. Here's what the acronym stands for:

S - Safety: Ground through all five of the senses and into earth (*Mulhadhara*).

E - Evoke: Connect to the memory, emotion, feeling (*Svadhistana*).

N - Notice: Observe the sensations and sacred messengers through the body (*Manipura*).

S - Sublimate: Decide what to do with the sensation - understand it, experience it, transform it, release it, expand it (*Anahata*).

F - Free: Express freely the sense or sensation through thought, journal, sound, creativity, conversation (*Vishuddha*).

U - Understand: See and accept with nonjudgment what these sacred messengers, sensations, and senses mean to you and where they may have come from (*Ajna*).

L - Love: Connect this inner revelation to higher power, intuition, and wisdom with love and compassion through affirmation (*Sahasrara*).

Your Sensual Saxophone

This can be done alone or with a partner, as a healing modality to bring more balance, energy, and awareness to the *chakras*. It can also be used while sitting opposite another, as well as during self-pleasure, foreplay, or sex - by one or both partners. You can set an intention when doing the practice. For a guided version, see the 'Sensual Self-Care Practice' in the Sensual Education Series, or 'The Breath of Ecstasy Tantric Date Night' for couples on the SOSA website (*see p.xxi*).

Here are the steps:

1. Create a sacred space where you feel comfortable and safe to express.

2. Lie down and breathe deeply.

3. Create a cycle with your breath, inhaling through your nose and exhaling through your mouth. Feel free to make sound and move your body.

4. Caress your whole body, noticing any sensations and emotions along the way.

5. Bring your fingertips or attention to each individual *chakra*, and bring your breath to circle in that center for a few minutes; change the depth of your breath, based on how you feel.

6. Bring your mind's eye to each *chakra*. Imagine the breath circulating there. You might see a color, the color of the *chakra*, a lotus unfolding, a swirling wheel, or a healing place in nature.

7. Connect the *chakras* and move from root to crown; begin to draw energy from the root, up the spine to the crown, over the head, and down the front of the body, to feed the energy back to the root, creating your own cocoon of healing energy. You can visualize this energy giving you all that your body, mind, and spirit need in this moment.

8. Complete the cycle and lie still in *savasana* (on your back) to integrate the experience.

9. To integrate, take time to journal, create art, or express your experience in conversation without judgment.

10. If with a partner, they can hold the time and place a gentle touch to caress and bring sensations to each *chakra*; their other palm can be underneath the body. Each partner can hold space for the other's healing and then swap, or both can do the breath together while seated or lying down.

Integration

1. Where do you feel pain/discomfort? What recurring medical problems do you experience? Can you relate these to your energy body or a specific *chakra*?

2. Which of your *chakras* feel balanced/strong?

3. Which of your *chakras* feel out of balance/weak?

4. Write down actions you can take to support balancing your *chakras*.

KEY TAKEAWAYS

~ The *nadis* are the network of channels, rivers, and reservoirs carrying energy through your body.

~ *Ida*, *pingala*, and *sushumna* are energetic pathways that can be used to transmute, transform, and expand our sensual energy.

~ The seven major *chakras* make up the Sensual Rivermap and correspond to energy centers along the spine, at the following locations: root, sacral center, solar plexus, heart, throat, third eye, and crown.

~ There are a variety of ways to balance, charge, unblock, and expand energy holistically — through yoga, breathwork, foods, activities, etc. — to keep your sensual river and energy body flowing so that sensation can be felt more deeply.

PART II

Your Nurtured Sensuality

Y ou are here not to learn how to be sensual, but to remove all the rocks in the river of sensuality that stop its currents from flowing through you. Sensuality is your nature. It is a reverse process to return to your true essence, your original sensual sacredness.

We are all innately sensual, yet over the course of our lives, through our experience in this lifetime and those of the generations that came before us, our sensuality is nurtured according to: who raises us; where we live; the norms of our country, culture, and society; as well as how our experience manifests in the body. In Part II, we'll explore the key blocks to sensuality I have discovered as themes running through the lives of the thousands of people from around the world we have served at SOSA. Then, we'll discover ways to move through these blocks and reconnect to our innate sensuousness!

From shame and trauma, to fear and stress – on the Tantric path, we are not here to label emotions, experiences, and sensations as good or bad or to rid ourselves of them. Instead, we are invited to experience them directly and subsequently weave them into the tapestry of living, so that we can live with deeper connection to our senses and awareness of how to express that more freely – be it through our work, intimacy, or creativity. Unlike many spiritual paths, Tantra is not about finding liberation in the next or afterlife. It is about living truly embodied: recognizing that *this* reality, *this* body, and *this* life itself is filled with potential, sacredness, and love.

For this reason, Tantra is sometimes known as the direct path[1] or as the path of nonduality, where we do not see ourselves as separate from our higher power, true essence, or divine nature. It is not about 'freeing' ourselves from suffering and negative traits; nor is it about bypassing or repressing them. It is about truly seeing reality as it is. Our sensuality, as we will see, is a spiritual pathway.

CHAPTER 5

Feeling Shame

Nurturing sensuality is a lifelong process that can be seriously blocked when we experience shame. Shame is one of the main obstacles to experiencing the full flow of our sensual energy through our body, mind, and spirit. Its often paralyzing effects can keep us from relishing in the innate beauty, pleasure, and sensuality available to each of us as humans.

In this chapter, we'll explore a method for digging into the deep and painful memories and experiences that underlie our shame — and we'll also discover that as we draw shame closer to ourselves, with compassion and care, it can be a powerful teacher coaxing us out of the need to conform to social norms, and instead to honor our own unique expression.

The Invisible Cloak of Shame

I recently dug up an old diary entry that helped me understand my relationship to shame before studying sensuality:

There are parts of myself I feel shame for. The parts which don't meet the status quo. The bits I can't shake. The bits which I could never tell my work. My family. My partner. All that is alive in me hides under a veil and sews itself a badge on the cloak of shame. It covers and hides me. And as I hide myself and offer only the crumbs of what remains, the selected parts, the good parts, the parts I think people will like, no one can truly know who I am. They connect only with the crumbs I offer them. The real me feels wrapped in a shell of invisibility, and not to be fully known or seen in this life — that is the real shame.

Over the years I have held space to explore sensuality, I've found shame is often one of the first sensations we bump into. Shame is a contraction, a hesitation, a withdrawal from the world and our interaction with it. It is an emotion that can have great control over us, the decisions we make, and how we choose to show up in the world. It can feel like a deep fear of exposure, or regret for past actions or experiences. It makes us feel like the possibility of exposing or expressing our true selves would mean an even deeper rejection of who we really are.

*Many of us have to create masks to wear in the world —
for our friends, family, work, culture, and society. Under
these masks is shame, which becomes a heavy cloak
that represses our senses, sensations, and sensuality,
and takes a lot of energy to uphold. To be anyone
other than who we truly are becomes exhausting.*

Shame dies when it is shared in spaces where we feel safe and accepted. This is often enough to begin to dispel the heavy sensational charge it can hold in our bodies. When we become more familiar with the sensation of shame, we might begin to follow its tail to the origin from which it stems and make an empowered choice as to whether we would like to remove its cloak or be more aware of when it appears. If we break the circuit of shame time and time again, we create space for new sensations that were blocked from emerging and find deeper sensuality, intimacy, and expression in our lives.

As we uncover shame that has calcified over our lifetime — physically, mentally, or energetically — we create space for sensual energy to flow through us and expand our awareness. This becomes a rich source of vitality, creativity, and confidence. Let's explore how to do that together.

Break the Shame Circuit

These are the steps we can take to break the circuit of shame:

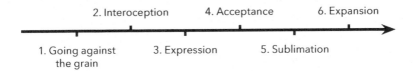

1. **Going against the grain:** norm + thought or action that goes against the norm

2. **Interoception:** experience of shame sensations + awareness of shame sensations

3. **Expression:** verbal or nonverbal expression of shameful thought, desire, or action

4. **Acceptance:** experience of acceptance of thought/desire

5. **Sublimation:** dispelling shame by releasing its charge of bodily sensation

6. **Expansion:** understanding the origin > peace/choice/action

What Is Shame?

Shame comes in many different shapes, forms, and sizes. For some, it feels like a flush of cheeks so red they could stop traffic; for others, a lump the size of a golf ball forms at the throat, mixed with a wish for an entire sinkhole to swallow us up.

Shame is something we all feel at some point in our lives, yet because our shame is not something we can easily share with others, it can be an incredibly isolating and uncomfortable internal experience. Although the degrees to which we feel shame vary, the very emotion itself – the fear of being found out, seen, heard, known – remains as human as breathing.

You may be wondering: *If it's so human, why do we feel shame?*

We feel hunger because we need to eat, we feel tired because we need to sleep, and we feel shame because we need to belong.

The word *shame* developed from the old English *scamu/sceomu*, which means not only 'guilt' or 'disgrace,' but also 'loss of esteem or reputation.' It evolved from the Germanic *scham/schande*, meaning both 'shame' and 'vulva.' Italian scholar Vittore Pisani pointed out the ancient Indo-European noun, *eskamitu*, meaning 'genitals,' and compared it to the Germanic word for *shame*. The roots of sensuality, sexuality, and shame are deeply intertwined through language, history, and society. Now, let's learn how to break its cycle.

Going Against the Grain

A philosopher named Hilge Landweer[1] from the Free University of Berlin created a study underpinning the conditions that must come together for us to feel shame.

▼ We must feel that we have transgressed a norm.

▼ We must view the norm as desirable or binding, because this is what makes transgressing it so uncomfortable.

▼ It isn't necessary for a disapproving person or group to be present; one's own critical thoughts are enough.

A *norm* refers to an agreed-upon set of behaviors and mindsets by a group that are considered usual, standard, typical, or expected. This will vary according to your friends, your family, your work, your religion, your culture, and the society around you.

By the time you're an adult, you'll have adopted a set of conscious and unconscious norms that determine the decisions you make and the way you live. As soon as you feel a thought or action that opposes that norm, you'll feel the uncomfortable sensation of shame in your body: a feeling of going against the grain. Your body was designed to do this, because as much as it needs to eat, breathe, and sleep to survive, it has been engineered by our evolution that it also needs to belong. When you feel shame, it's your sense of belonging to your tribe that is at threat.

A study from Harvard University[2] found that, contrary to what most people think, it's not career achievement, exercise, or a healthy diet that's the key to a long, healthy life. Instead, people who are connected to their family, friends, and community are happier and physically healthier than those who are less connected. Connection, belonging, and being a part of something determine the quality and quantity of our life. This connection comes from sharing ourselves, our highs, our lows, our vulnerability, and sometimes even our shame, with others.

You are not alone in feeling shame. Shame has evolved to deliver you a message: that what you may be thinking, doing, or thinking of doing could lead to a sense of exclusion from your 'pack' and consequently affect your overall well-being.

Interoception

Along with the five senses we explored in Part I of the book, there are subtler senses. Interoception is one of these lesser-known but important senses on our journey to sensuality. It is the sense that helps us understand and feel what's going on inside the body, which can be both conscious and unconscious.

Interoception is the ability to sense internal signals in the body. For example, the sensations of when we're hungry and when we need to go to the toilet are taught to us in our earliest days. Other sensations — like what happens when we feel shame, stress, or fear — are less well taught but can be brought into the field of our awareness. Just like linking the sensations of when we are thirsty with getting a glass of water, we can link the sensations of shame with awareness of contraction, hesitation, or rejection — and then take action to accept, empathize, and understand these sensations.

Connect to your interoception. Pause, close your eyes, and think for a moment about how shame feels in your body. Where are the sensations? Charles Darwin attributed the flushing of the face, rush of blood to the cheeks, downcast eyes, slackened posture, and lowered head as the physiological sign of internal shame. Collapsing the body is our inner signal to withdraw from interactions that could threaten our belonging. If we were to interact or be found out, the sensation of shame in our body can feel like a life-or-death situation.

Among our ancient ancestors, exclusion might mean being left behind outside our cave while predators lurked, or not receiving a ration of the food shared among our group. In the modern era, exclusion usually looks like a social threat but can still feel like a survival threat. This is because shame is connected to the limbic system, a set of structures in the brain that are responsible for our behavioral and emotional responses, especially concerning survival, reproduction, and caring for our young. It's also connected to our 'fight or flight' threat response. Once the limbic system is triggered, the set of uncomfortable bodily responses will ensue.

The discomfort of shame could also be an opportunity to discover the parts of ourselves that were shaped by our belonging to a particular group – whether our family, politics, religion, race, media, or culture. We might find the submerged aspects of ourselves that long to be seen – the self underneath the shame that longs to be known. We get to open the door to see ourselves and the motherboard that drives our daily interactions, our wishes and our desires, with greater clarity. The iceberg under the surface that runs the show begins to emerge.

It's a voyage that often feels like a terrifying and grave departure from the self, but when we experience the sensations of our shame with awareness rather than pushing them deeper into the unconscious, we are able to draw aspects of our thoughts, desires, or actions closer, to reveal who we truly are underneath social constructs.

Expression

The expression of shame may first come as the revelation of the thought underneath the sensation. To give it a channel to move from repression is the healing balm of expression. Expression can be both verbal and nonverbal. It can be the conversation you have with your mind and your body: 'I see this shame I have about the hair on my body because of...' or 'I see this shame I have about sensuality because...'

Expression can occur through journaling, playing music, making art, or moving your body to express the script emerging from the shame. Other forms of expression include spoken word in a space or group where you feel nonjudgment and acceptance. This provides a channel for the shame to emerge from repression.

In the Shakti Circle, an online community space at SOSA, we gather with people from around the world to take off the masks, break taboos, and go on journeys of personal unraveling through interoception, connection, and expansion. I have noticed an incredible pattern: that when the first brave soul takes off the mask and shares their story, the kind they would never tell their friends or family, it opens the pathway for others to step out of the shadows and share their experience.

The last person to share in the Shakti Circle often rounds off with, 'I never thought I would say this, but here goes...' This creates an opportunity to experience expressing our truth, perhaps for the first time, and reprogram our nervous system to find that sharing won't disconnect us from our human tribe; we won't die or be left out of the cave. As a receiver, we experience connection and resonance through the stories of others. This becomes a practice and template for our lives outside the circle.

To offer some insight into the Shakti Circle, these are stories we've collected over the years that offer a light into the soul beyond the crumbs of shame. I want to thank anyone who has attended our circle, which is the heart of the SOSA community. The stories have been made anonymous and mixed with other stories to respect the privacy of our attendees. As you read, cast judgment aside, connect your eyes with your heart, and engage with the courage and vulnerability of the people who've shared.

Tanya's Story: Hair and Hiding

For as long as Tanya can remember, she's felt shame about the hair on her body. When she was a child, it was a soft, fuzzy line that joined her eyebrows and extended down her arms and legs. She wasn't aware of it until someone on the school playground pointed it out with remarks she replayed in her head until her adulthood.

She recalls going home after school, mortified. She opened the bathroom cabinet and reached for her father's razor. She took the blade straight down the center of her face, leaving the ends of her eyebrows barely intact. She burned in the rash of shame it left her with. No matter how much she plucked, tweezed, and removed the hair, the shame from the playground lived in her face and body.

As she grew older, she wore a fringe, covered her body, and avoided eye contact. She didn't want to be seen or touched. The cloak of shame wrapped its arms around her and developed into body dysmorphia. The moment she shared this in the circle, she was met with love, connection, and acceptance for the first time. The practice we shared sparked a new relationship with her body.

Kara's Story: Regrets and Sexual Health

Kara suffered a heartbreak after her partner cheated on her. It felt like her whole world was falling apart. Not knowing how to handle the pain, disappointment, rejection, and loss she was feeling, she started engaging in casual sexual encounters with people she met at nightclubs.

One day, blisters broke out around her vulva. She went to the doctor and was told she had contracted herpes. Later, that week she received results from another STI test saying that she had chlamydia. While she could treat chlamydia, she felt the herpes virus was full of shame she could never share with anyone. She felt so alone.

She came to SOSA 10 years after the diagnosis. In this time, she had never told anyone or sought help. As she connected the dots of her experience, she began to view her journey with empathy, realizing she was not alone. She began to feel more confident approaching the conversation in new relationships.

Pamela's story: Religion and Wrongness

Pamela grew up in a very religious household. She had broken away from the religion in her early 30s and was now in her 50s. During a circle, Pamela ran into the shame she had encountered around the body. She had learned that pleasure was a sin and that enjoying the sensory world was not in line with the 'good' moral values of her upbringing or culture.

Although she had left the religion, she realized that the block she was holding between herself and deeper sensuality had been ingrained in her childhood religious classes. She hadn't realized the impact it was having on the way she was experiencing her body, relationships, and intimacy until now.

As she shared, she met others who'd had a similar experience. Newly empowered, she decided to embark on a gentle exposure to sensuality, with regular practices to distinguish sex and shame from sensuality.

It all seems so easy when we read about these experiences. But how do we lift the cloak if we can't find our Shakti Circle around us? Fear not: Tantra has some more incredible goddesses for that!

Acceptance

When we feel shame, approval and acceptance may not need to come from others or external validation. Tantra offers us the progressive path of gradually working with our shadows. It offers us deity meditation that has the power to untangle blocks such as shame, fear, trauma, and stress, which keep us from knowing our true divine and sensuous nature.

Many Tantric deities have fierce, shocking, and sometimes repulsive[3] appearances, and aren't your average 'beautiful' goddess. They instead represent all the parts within ourselves we may repress. This calls forth the transformative power of self-acceptance and puts us in touch with our own *shakti* nature. We recognize that we're exactly the way the divine wants to express herself through us.

Deities reflect aspects of nature and our own psyche that can be contacted as personalities or presences, either externally or internally.[4] Instilling this aspect of the *shakti* consciousness within ourselves can become an incredibly transformative route to shift shame and accept our wholeness from within.

Archetypes are universal symbols, motifs, or characters that reveal the hidden patterns underneath our choices and point us toward universal human motivations. They appear as figures and themes across the arts, literature, mythology, and religion, and appear across different cultures and historical eras. Examples are the maiden, mother, crone, and hag, or the joker, hero, and villain we see in so many movies and stories.

Although the term is as old as storytelling itself, Swiss psychiatrist Carl Jung brought the concept of *archetypes* into psychology in 1919 with his paper 'Instinct and the unconscious.'[5] He described archetypes as primordial patterns that stem from the 'collective' unconscious, or the layer of the unconscious that is beyond the individual and a part of the common collective. He saw the collective unconscious as a source of empowerment.

As we make these connections and draw a bridge between the conscious and the unconscious, archetypes offer us an opportunity to present our shame, experience resonance, and move toward acceptance of our sensual essence.

Sally Kempton shares how in the Tantric tradition:

> ...deity meditation gives us access to a power that works on a deeper level than is available through conventional psychology; the transformative power of the goddess energies can untangle psychic knots, calling forth specific transformative forces within the mind and heart.[6]

The goddess-consorts are seen as embodying the power and active energy of the male gods; both are interdependent aspects of reality – the unmanifest and the manifest, the conscious and the unconscious. It is the goddesses and their *shakti* that activate the functions of the male god figures.

Brahma is the creator god who brings the world into manifestation through the personification of his *shakti*, Saraswati, the goddess of creativity. Vishnu is the god of preservation and protection, and his *shakti* and power is Lakshmi, the goddess of abundance and nourishment. Shiva is the god of destruction and lord of Yoga and Tantra; his *shakti* is encompassed by the goddesses Durga, Parvati, and Kali. Behind all of these stand Mahadevi, the great goddess who gives life to all the other deities, as well as the power to perform their cosmic roles.

This leads us to the Tantric goddesses known as the Dasa Mahavidyas. *Dasa* translates from Sanskrit as 'ten,' *maha* means 'great,' and *vidya* means 'knowledge,' with each one being a path unto herself. These are the 10 great wisdom goddesses, or cosmic personalities. The Mahavidyas can be found in many ancient texts. They became central to Shaktism, a spiritual school of thought in which the supreme cosmic energy known as *adi parashakti* was envisaged as Mahadevi, the great primordial goddess. Although there is one pervasive Shakti, the Dasa Mahavidyas represent her 10 different facets.[7]

> *As you align with the energies of the Mahavidya goddesses in this chapter, you'll begin to make decisions that are in alignment with your spirit: You'll take lovers and lovemaking experiences that are in orgasmic alignment; you'll make a career move that's in dharmic alignment; and you'll be able to resonate with the energetic frequency of the goddess archetypes you're attracted to.*

In his book *Tantric Visions of the Divine Feminine: The Ten Mahavidyas*, David Kinsley reminds us of a theme across the mythological stories that surround the Mahavidyas: That is, these goddesses assert their independence from their husbands (usually Shiva). They are not just consorts — they take center stage. Uma Dinsmore-Tuli shares how they can also be mapped to the different stages of cyclical wisdom and life.[8]

They can draw us to find courage, independence from attachments, and the ability to weave together parts of ourselves we may find difficult to acknowledge or accept. They welcome home all the misfit parts of ourselves we have submerged, failed to acknowledge, or cast away in shame or repression. In seeing that all these aspects are also in the Mahavidyas, we're invited to consider that they're not separate from us and have the power to uproot shame.

The Dasa Mahavidyas

In the *Tantras*, goddesses have three forms with which we can engage. They have beautiful visual form in sculptures and paintings; sacred geometrical forms known as *yantras* (which are regarded as containing each goddess); as well as *bija mantras* that carry them through sound.[9] The *mantras* are usually instructed to be shared under guidance of a teacher due to the energy, shifts, and power they can invoke.

There are individual mythologies for the goddesses, too. Each of the goddesses has her own *siddhi*, or special power, which I share on the following pages through an individual message from the deity. I am also adding a sensual archetype for each Mahavidya, for our own explorations in this book.

Most of us have more than one archetype alive within our personalities, and many of them will change as we venture through different periods of our lives. It is not only women who have relationships with the goddesses and their *shakti*, but all humans, no matter what gender. You can see which Mahavidya calls out to you most at different times in your life and work with her messages of empowerment.

If you experience your sensuality one way your entire life, you might wish to play with different archetypes. For example, a queen might have an energy different to a sacred temple dancer, and a warrior will have an energy different to a maiden. Choose an evening to go out and embody this energy with yourself or in play with a partner. Think how the Mahavidya you've selected would think, speak how they would speak, walk how they would walk, and act as they would act. Use your intuition and think of it as spiritual roleplay – where you get to expand your sensual awareness beyond who you are!

Kali

The dark goddess of transformation

I empower you to face the fear, endings and darkness to bring forth the parts of you that are ready to change and transform, so you can experience new beginnings. (We'll learn more about Kali in Chapter 7.)

Sensual archetype: Mother

Tara

The goddess who compassionately guides and protects through difficulty

I empower you to drop the labels society has given you, to see clearly your true nature.

Sensual archetype: Friend next door

Tripura Sundari/Shodashi

The goddess of the three worlds/the 16-year-old goddess

I empower you to move through attachments, expectations, cravings, and addictions to connect to your deepest needs, playfulness, and desires.

Sensual archetype: Maiden

Bhuavaneśhvari

The goddess whose body is the world

I empower you to drop self-criticism and self-loathing, and I remind you of the power of love and beauty within yourself and the natural world.

Sensual archetype: Mystic

Bhairavi

The goddess of fierceness

I empower you to face all that disgusts you, and embrace your anger and rage, transforming them into deeper self-acceptance of yourself and others.

Sensual archetype: Boss

Chinnamasta

The self-decapitated goddess of sex

I empower you to move from shame to embrace your sexual energy as a form of self-empowerment, creativity, and healing.

Sensual archetype: Wild woman

Dhumavati

The widow goddess

I empower you to release fears of being alone and aging to embrace the wisdom in each day as you grow older.

Sensual archetype: Wise crone

Bagalamukhi

The paralyzing goddess

I empower you to paralyze the enemies of your mind and thoughts that block you from knowing who you truly are, as I guide you toward your inner teacher.

Sensual archetype: Warrior

Matangi

The outcast creative goddess

I empower you to go beyond what is 'normal' and embrace the full weirdness, strangeness, and uniqueness of who you are, even if it's different.

Sensual archetype: Creative artist

Kamalatmika

The goddess of pleasure and delight

I empower you to release feelings of unworthiness and low self-esteem to experience the beauty, pleasure, and abundance in the everyday.

Sensual archetype: Queen

▼ Activity ▼

Mahavidya Meditation

This meditation will help you to overcome shame and invoke the guidance and connect to the qualities of the Mahavidya goddess you are calling in. Allow 20-30 minutes for this practice.

1. Set aside five minutes to move your body (through dancing, shaking, or yoga).

2. Lie down and close your eyes. Allow 10 minutes to go through each part of your body, relaxing it along the way.

3. For 10-15 minutes, imagine yourself in a beautiful place in nature. It's nighttime. As you look up, you sense the divine feminine Shakti of the natural world. As you breathe in and bathe in her presence, she begins to come closer.

4. Imagine your own presence of the goddess you are calling in, or use the images on the SOSA website (see p.xxi). As she emerges, she gazes into your eyes with complete love and acceptance. She sees your gifts, your shame, your fear, your trauma, your blocks, your mistakes, your regrets - she sees everything you hide, and she still loves, accepts, and holds you.

5. Connect your breath from your heart to hers. With each breath, draw in her presence and let it flow through your body. And with each exhale, let go of whatever needs to be released. As you inhale, you draw in love and acceptance; as you exhale, you release shame, fear, trauma, stress, and anything else that does not serve you.

Sublimation

In science, sublimation is the process of turning one substance into another. In Tantra, this same process is used to alchemize sensations and emotions in the body. When you experience the sensation, express it, and feel acceptance; this helps you to discharge the often heavy and overwhelming sensations of shame from the body.

Imagine your shoulders squeezed up to your ears, a lump in your throat, and butterflies in your stomach. Feel yourself slowly releasing this through your awareness and expression.

A powerful space to sublimate energy is the heart center. Bring your awareness of all your sensations to your heart with a deep breath, and transform them with a new affirmation of acceptance, love, and acknowledgment. Some examples of affirmations are:

▼ I see who I am beyond the shame I feel about...

▼ I accept who I am with love and compassion.

▼ I am love consciousness and the expression of Shakti manifesting herself.

Expansion

Once we have followed all the steps of this process, we create a new awareness of how shame manifests in the body. Every time we experience shame or choose not to avoid it, we take steps to break its cycle. When we are caught in its cycle, we cannot unravel the true thought, wish, or person underneath our shame.

As the sensation of shame begins to feel less overwhelming, we might also explore the questions of its origin: *What norm is this breaking? Where did I learn this norm? What would happen if I broke the cycle and experienced something beyond it?*

Empowered with this knowledge, we can then make an informed choice as to how we'd like to proceed, with a sense of expansion.

▼ Activities ▼

Nyasa – Infusing the Body with the Divine

This is a Tantric practice that involves infusing the body with the divine, which helps to break patterns of shame and rewire the body with new, conscious awareness. I thank Whitney Wheelock of the Kaula Tantra Tradition for introducing me to this.

Traditionally, the practice is shared by chanting each letter in the Sanskrit alphabet. Each letter is considered a divine *mantra* and correlates to a part of the body; the pronunciation is important and can be found on the SOSA website.

Another way to do this is to pass through each area of the body with your deep presence or touch while chanting *aham devi*, which means 'I am divine/goddess/Shakti/power.'

If doing this in a pair or group, you can say: 'This is the beautiful X of Y.' X is the body part you can apply gentle touch and awareness to, and Y is the name of the person being touched. This way, areas that hold shame will be infused with this new script and divine energy.

Break the Cycle Using the SENSFUL Method

It is important to take your time with each SENSFUL step. Only move forward when you feel ready to. If any strong emotions arise, complete the cycle of feeling them, and express this by moving, sounding, and freeing any stuck energy, to attune to yourself from a place of love and healing rather than judgment.

1. **S - Safety:** Find a comfortable place to call your own. Sit down and take a few minutes to arrive by connecting to your five senses.

2. **E - Evoke:** Write down a story of shame you have experienced in your life.

3. **N - Notice:** Take note of where you feel the sensations of shame in your body.

4. **S - Sublimate:** Rub your hands to create warmth, and touch the area. Notice if any new thoughts arise. Breathe deeply, allowing the shame to be seen and felt.

5. **F - Free:** Express what is coming up for you, either verbally or by journaling.

6. **U - Understand:** Follow the trail of the shame, and journal about where this shame may have arisen from.

7. **L - Love:** Repeat words of affirmation as shared in the previous exercise and send them through your whole body.

Shakti Circle Using the SENSFUL Method

Spaces of belonging, reflection, and expressing your true, authentic self are key to moving through shame and toward wholeness. Find a local circle near you, join our online Shakti Circles at SOSA, or create your own circle using the following steps. The circle is an equal space, with no hierarchy, even for the person holding the space. You can invite a few people to gather around the moon cycle or once a month, to explore, share, and express themselves on different subjects.

1. **S - Safety:** Open by setting an intention/theme and introduce the circle framework (nonjudgment, freedom, confidentiality,

etc.). Offer an opening ritual, such as lighting a candle to open the space. Finally, offer a practice, such as grounding, to arrive in the space and body.

2. **E - Evoke:** Guide a journey based on the topic or theme, such as shame. This could be a visualization, meditation, movement, creative activity, or any skill you'd like to share and explore.

3. **N - Notice:** Guide participants to notice the sensations before, during, and after the practice. Offer journaling questions to reflect on the practice, setting a time to return together to process the experience and sensations.

4. **S - Sublimate:** Offer another practice to shift the sensations into love, aliveness, and awareness; this could be eye gazing, shaking, dancing, or yoga.

5. **F - Free:** Open the sharing space, reminding people of the guidelines to connect eyes and ears with heart and listen without advice or judgment. Set a time limit and focus on one of the journaling questions to keep the flow of the circle. The space holder can thank each person for sharing, or mirror back what has been said with affirmation. The other circle members can offer gestures of understanding, such as placing a hand on the heart if they have felt this, too, or writing in the chat box if online.

6. **U - Understand:** Reflect on any themes that arose from hearing others' stories and add any understanding to your own story or journey. If there are any actions you can take from this understanding, you can journal about it or discuss.

7. **L - Love:** Together, finish with a universal affirmation of gratitude – for each other, for yourselves, and/or for the practices you've shared, through a *mantra*, a song, a prayer, or a dance.

Integration

1. What norms have you gone against, based on your family, friends, society, religion, or culture?

2. Are there any parts of your body where you feel shame or that you hide? Notice where this might stem from.

3. Notice which of the Mahavidyas you might be resonating with right now, and which ones you'd like to explore.

4. Try one of the practices to work with shame and reflect on your findings.

Key Takeaways

~ We feel shame any time we go against the norms that emerge from culture, society, and family.

~ Shame stems from the instinctive human need to belong.

~ Shame is a cycle that can be broken through awareness of the norm transgressed, interoception, expression, acceptance, sublimation, and expansion.

~ The Shakti Circle provides a powerful, nonjudgmental space for exploring and expressing shame, and for realizing that we are not alone in our experiences.

~ Exploring archetypes such as the Mahavidyas (Tantric wisdom goddesses) can be powerful ways of emulating divine qualities, empowering ourselves, and finding acceptance within – especially when it comes to integrating qualities we may have disowned.

CHAPTER 6

Feeling Trauma

Trauma and sensuality are not often associated or seen in the same sentence together, yet they are experienced in the same body and share a unique relationship. In this chapter, we'll examine the link between trauma and our sensuality through the lens of psychology and Tantra. We'll dive into what happens in the body when we are experiencing trauma, and what we can do to heal trauma that stops us from experiencing deeper sensuality.

Tracing Trauma Backwards

Growing up, I had a best friend and cousin sister, Jalpa, to whom this book is dedicated. She was murdered a few days before my 10th birthday; this was followed by the illnesses and deaths of three close family members each year until I was 14.

By the time I was in my early twenties, I had so many questions that my law degree and Western education couldn't answer — questions I had suppressed into numbness to block the feelings these difficult experiences brought up, which kept me from feeling anything at all. But I had a deep longing in my bones to know what it really meant to die, and in turn, what it meant to live for this short and undisclosed time we get to spend here, in this body and on this planet. My questioning heart and numb body, which occasionally raced at the thought of these losses, are what led me back home, to India.

Each morning in my motherland, the birds called and roosters crowed loudly. I pulled my head from the hard pillows in my uncle's house and felt my feet touch the cold tile floor. You could hear the clattering of chai pots, roar of indigo-colored gas flames, ringing of temple bells in the distance, and bicycle chains zipping nearby. For months, we gathered in a small room in the basement of a local yoga teacher, Manjuben. There were no mirrors or music in the room, no crystals or yoga leggings. Instead, the room filled with people wearing Indian yoga clothes — cotton trousers and long *kurta* tops — and woven woolen yoga mats known as *asana*.

In this class, there were postures, in addition to meditation, *mantras*, *pranayama*, and *kriyas* (cleansing techniques). Instructions were direct and without jokes, fluff, or metaphors. The sequences took us through physical, energetic, and spiritual realms. The postures repeated daily as we sank deeper and deeper into them.

Was this the true yoga? I wondered.

Around one month into consistent daily practice, I discovered that certain postures would leave me in a flood of tears. Holding certain muscle groups caused my heart to flutter. Stepping off the mat, I started to hear certain words that would make my palms sweat. Some *mantras* brought a lump to my throat, filled with intense emotions, and other breath patterns brought flashes of memories I'd kept stuffed down for years. It was the first time I could feel the emotional and physical pain in my body. The practices were allowing me to experience and close the cycles I had kept looping in my nervous system for years. A sense of home, healing, and safety was being restored. Each day of practice provided a gentle pathway for numbness to transform into sensation, and for that sensation to integrate and transform my life.

After several years of study, I learned that traditional Eastern systems of embodiment are not systems of discussion but of practice. You do the practice and you feel the result; there is little opportunity for discussion after this. Yet, growing up in the West, I yearned for the words to process what was unraveling in my body.

I came back to the UK with a few more questions in my mind around the integration of traumatic experiences that are processed through the body using somatic practices and frameworks of safety and integration. I studied a foundation of art therapy and later began clinical psychotherapy training for individuals and couples, where I could learn more about therapeutically informed spaces for healing and make use of the content that emerged from the practices with my clients. (I am eternally grateful to my own therapist, TH, whom I've learned so much with and from over the past several years.)

Although the Eastern and Western systems of healing were built independently, I found the drawing together of their tools offered a unique recipe, encompassing the fact that we're not just this body and not just this mind — we're whole beings made of mind, body, and spirit, undergoing the human experience of living. This is the recipe, bridging the Eastern embodiment and Western therapeutic frameworks, I now share at SOSA.

What Is Trauma?

Imagine a filing system for your memories. Each memory is created, stored, and then closed, ready for opening when we want to remember or recall a story to our friends or family. We have folders for each year of our lives. Some memories are stored in images that run through our mind; others are stored in sensations, smells, sounds, and senses.

An ex-lover's perfume may bring back a flash of a person we haven't thought about in years. A particular taste will take us right back to the childhood dining table with a grandparent. A traumatic memory can feel like a file has opened, but its papers are flying around – sometimes illegible, hard to catch hold of, and even more difficult to know how to close. Amidst all the chaos, memories from traumatic events can often become distorted. This can feel like sudden flashbacks, cloudiness, panic, heart palpitations, and triggers that catch us off guard, catalyzed by the senses.

The word *trauma* stems from the Greek word meaning to 'wound' or 'pierce.' While some physical wounds can be seen in manifest form, in the bandage on our leg or the scar on our arms, emotional wounds are often unseen by the naked eye, even as they pierce the inner world. Certain senses can open the wound and bring us viscerally back to the moment they happened, as if they were happening again. Some wounds stay open – like a scab that doesn't heal and keeps us looping in cycles of fear that infect our enjoyment of life. Such wounds might feel so normal, they often go untreated, unacknowledged, and unhealed while they remain open inside of us. This is because they're not something we see — they're something we feel or sense, as individuals and as racial groups, genders, sexualities, and entire cultures and societies.[1]

Dr. Rick Bradshaw defines trauma as occurring when something negative and unexpected happens that leaves us feeling confused, overwhelmed, and powerless.[2] It can stem from the experience of serious harm, death, or injury, to any everyday experience of distress, fear, or helplessness concerning ourselves or another. It could happen once or over a series of experiences repeated over a period of time.

Whether we are aware of it or not, trauma communicates through messengers of sensation, such as contraction and relaxation, pain and comfort, constriction and expansion, numbness and energy. It drives how we experience life, the decisions we make, and of course, how we experience our sensuality — often without our knowledge. Trauma's primary concern is our survival, and the same way we flip through these pages, it too flips through the stories it's collected through our life and genetics to inform us of what is safe and what isn't.

Our bodies hold countless wordless stories,
with history written down our spines and
experiences carried through our cells.

In yogic and Tantric philosophy, this is explored through the concept of *samskaras,* mental impressions or recollections stored in the unconscious through past experiences or thoughts over a long period of time. They could also be passed down through generational history and previous lifetimes. *Samskaras* are mirrored in our thoughts, habits, decisions, and patterns. Some *samskaras* will sprout like seeds that align us with our truth, purpose, and heart; other *samskaras* are like weeds that draw a veil between us and our true nature, to create separation, contraction, and fear. They give rise to *vasanas,* which are the wordless impressions arising from past experiences that form the basis for who we think we are. [3] All our actions, thoughts, and *samskaras* are brought forward, from one year to the next, one generation to the next, and possibly one lifetime to the next.

Trauma can affect us as individuals and also as communities, as it can be passed down intergenerationally, through our genetics or the societies and cultures in which we live. There is no set standard for what is considered a trauma; it is defined more by what happened to the person experiencing it, and is unique to each individual according to their physical, mental, social, and emotional makeup.

Most trauma, whether isolated or complex,
individual or collective, from our personal lived
experiences or intergenerational, stems from
events that are usually beyond our control and can
result in lasting impacts that affect our internal
world, our relationships, and our sensuality.

So, what happens inside of us when we experience trauma — and how do we work through it?

Completing the Process

When I was in Botswana in 2022, I witnessed the chase of predators and prey for the first time. After the prey speeds across the barren sand in the race for its life and stands still in its tracks once the threat has passed, it shakes, trembles, coos, grunts, and makes sounds. When it completes this process, it goes off on its way. This allows the animal to discharge the high level of hormones released in its bloodstream and brings the cycle of fight/flight/freeze to a close. There is a clear beginning, middle, and end to the process. Trauma is stored in the body when the cycle is incomplete, and the residue of the sensations continues to be felt in the body, as if it were happening again in the here and now.

While it was once thought that trauma is a purely mental process, ancient Eastern systems and the latest Western research have gone on to uncover that trauma affects the whole body. Most notably, Bessel van der Kolk's *The Body Keeps the Score*[4] and Peter Levine's *Waking the Tiger*[5] underpinned and revolutionized the way the West thinks about the impact of trauma, and helped to understand better how we can work somatically with its heavy burden in the body.

So, what's happening in the body when we experience trauma? Our autonomic nervous system creates a response that produces the stress chemicals cortisol and adrenalin, to prepare the body for the potential emergency that might threaten its safety or survival. This affects the vagus nerve, which is also referred to as the wandering nerve – or, as Resmaa Menakem calls it, the *soul nerve*, because it is the mind/body connector.[6] It connects the brainstem, pharynx, heart, lungs, stomach, gut, cervix, and spine. When activated, this might mean a rise in blood pressure, heart rate, and sweating, as well as change of breath and dilation of the pupils.

During this time, other bodily functions – such as digestion, immunity, and sex drive – are suppressed. Things such as eating, enjoying the sensory world, or seeking a mate to procreate with take a back seat to the body's survival.

Stephen Porges's polyvagal theory[7] gives us an understanding of the vagus nerve's role in helping us regulate our emotions and fear response. He notes that the autonomic nervous system regulates three fundamental physiological instincts, which are determined by how unsafe the environment feels.

1. The first instinct is to turn to social engagement, where we might shout, call for help, or seek support from those around us.

2. The second instinct is to fight or flee; our body produces the adrenalin and stress hormones to attack or quickly run from the threat.

3. The third instinct is to freeze or collapse, which kicks in if we can't fight or escape, and have no other choice but to play dead, preserve our energy, and shut down our systems until the threat has passed.

Trauma is not just the isolated event or ongoing incidents we experience, but the 'wounding' or 'piercing' we continue to experience from its incomplete process inside us. This can affect us on a physical, mental, spiritual, and sensual level. Physically, the stress chemicals released to save us from the threat get stuck, making it feel like we're in a continued or easily triggered state of high alert or still frozen in the experience. In our minds, the content of the traumatic event can get mixed up or lost, causing us to forget the details of what happened, in order to survive. When we are trying to survive, mentally or physically, sensuality takes a back seat.

Pierre Janet was a French psychologist, physician, philosopher, and psychotherapist who specialized in the way traumatic memories are stored. He coined the term *dissociation*,[8] a state that prevents trauma from integrating within the memory. This means it becomes split or dual – and the thoughts, energy, emotions, and sensations of the event are stored separately, frozen and mostly incomprehensible. The dissociated person finds it difficult to remember or know the difference between whether the event happened in the past, the present, or the future. Imagine the papers from the filing cabinet have landed disorganized, back to front, and illegible.

If a traumatic event can't be remembered with words or verbal language, psychoanalytic thought suggests it will likely be acted out or repeated in other ways. For example, a child who has a parent or guardian with addictions may unconsciously go on to find a partner with addictions. Also, according to a study exploring the hidden impact behind crimes, more than 51 percent of adults who were abused as children experienced domestic abuse later in life.[9] This shows us how important it is to process trauma and close its cycles in our physical, mental, emotional, sensual, and spiritual inner landscape, so we can heal and move forward. What is not worked through can be repeated, as the cellular energy and process are still open and seeking completion through our *vasanas*.

As I've discovered with any embodiment practices that use the wisdom of the body to release trauma from unprocessed experiences, emotions, and memories, it's helpful to process what comes up with a compassionate and experienced psychotherapist, which can provide a regular and safe container in which to explore the material. I wholeheartedly believe in both body-based and mind-based practices for the treatment of trauma.

Layers, Knots, and Locks of Trauma

The Tantra Yoga system sees the body in a multidimensional way, which is helpful for the treatment and healing of trauma. The *Taittiriya Upanishad* describes the body as being made up of five distinct layers, much like the layers of an onion, known as the *koshas*.

The Pancha *Koshas*: The Five Casings

A *kosha* translates to a 'sheath' or 'casing' because each fits into the next like a Russian nesting doll. This system means we not only work with the physical body, but all the layers within us that may be affected by trauma, to bring us back to our core, known as *anandamaya* – or our bliss nature. There are five *koshas* we'll explore here.

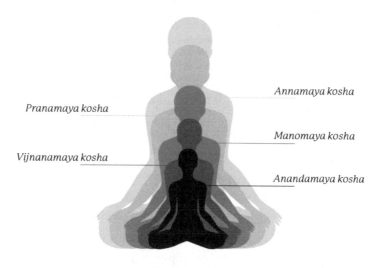

Pranamaya kosha

Vijnanamaya kosha

Annamaya kosha

Manomaya kosha

Anandamaya kosha

The five *koshas*

Annamaya kosha

This is the physical layer comprising the manifest, physical body. Any impacts on the inner *koshas* will filter through and impact this outermost layer, and vice versa, the same way a root's health will show in its fruits and flowers. This is the physical impact of trauma.

Pranamaya kosha

This is the vital life force or energetic layer. The flow of *prana* is as important as the blood flowing through our veins. Where trauma is stored and *prana* is blocked in the body's *nadis* (energy channels), it will manifest in the *annamaya kosha* or physical layer as discomfort, pain, inflammation, numbness, or disease.

Manomaya kosha

This is the mental layer. As though they were messengers, the thoughts in our mind affect the *prana* that flows around our body, and vice versa. The story of the trauma can loop through our thoughts. Our thoughts interweave and feed the outer *pranamaya* and *annamaya koshas*.

Vijnanamaya kosha

This is the intuitive layer. It's the part of ourselves underneath the thinking mind that's able to witness our thoughts and experience the self as separate from them. It's the pause between the thoughts and the stillness between the breath that leads us to experience this layer. In other words, it's awareness itself.

Anandamaya kosha

This is the bliss layer. It's the core experience of unconditional love, joy, and bliss. Beyond the witnessing mind, we dissolve separation, the ego, and the I-self, so this bliss can be fully experienced. We don't see ourselves as experiencing bliss when we're in this layer. We *are* bliss itself. This bliss is perceived through the states or glimpses of oneness, where we reach *atman* – the experience of our eternal soul, connection with our higher power, and the divine essence of the universe.

When trauma is experienced and the cycle isn't completed, it may get stored in the physical, energetic, and mental layers, and block access to the *vijnanamaya* and *anandamaya koshas*. Trauma can be felt in the knots and tangles that exist in different parts of the body. These knots are known as *granthis*. The *granthis* are physical, energetic, and psychic contractions that stop the free flow of sensual life force and energy in the *nadis*. The *granthis* block our *chakras* and stop *kundalini shakti*, the sensual and sexual energy, from rising. This keeps us from pleasure, healing, creativity, connection, and spiritual evolution. In the West, these knots are generally referred to as *body armoring*.

In Tantra Yoga and Tantric bodywork, we work with practices to invoke *kundalini shakti* so it can freely course through the body. As it does so, it'll begin to highlight knots of numbness, pain, trauma, or discomfort. When the practitioner or bodyworker attends to the knots, any numbness will turn to pain and any pain will turn to sensation, where sensation begins to be felt, nutrient-rich oxygenated blood and energy are flowing, and sensual healing is happening. In this process, the suppressed emotions, trauma, and memories may unravel in order to complete the process that's stored or repeating in the body and psyche.

It's important to provide or allow space for these emotional cycles to complete, and for the person practicing or receiving to know they can experience the memory or emotional response safely in their body. This allows the client to complete and break the looping trauma cycle in the cells.[10] Processing what has come up after the session, whether with a therapist or bodyworker, allows the client to pluck the paper flying around in the air and file it properly in their memory, as well as discharge the energy and repeating patterns from the trauma through the layers of their body.

Depending on where trauma is stored in the body, there may be different *granthis* around the body that can be unknotted through Tantra Yoga, Tantric bodywork, or the *bandhas* and practices at the end of this chapter.

There are three key *granthis* to know:

1. **Brahma granthi** is a tangle of energetic channels sitting in the pelvis and genitals. This is around the area of *Mulhadhara*. When energy knots here, it can evoke feelings of addiction, lack, threat, trauma, and fear. It symbolizes survival, sex, safety, instinct, and desire.

2. **Vishnu granthi**, located between the heart *chakra* and the solar-plexus *chakra*, is a knot that creates contractions through dependent attachments, grief, ego, and power play. This attachment can make us feel alone, separated, and disconnected from ourselves, others, and the world around us.

3. **Rudra granthi** is located between the throat and center of the forehead, or *Vishuddha* and *Ajna chakras*. It governs mental patterns, thoughts, or stories that block sensual and sexual energy from rising to the crown and connecting us to our higher power.

Bandhas for Energy Leakage

Bandhas translates to 'locks' that directly work to pierce through the three *granthis* we explored in this chapter. Please do not undertake these locks if you are pregnant, have anything in your pelvis such as a coil/tampon/baby/menstruation, or have high blood pressure or any medical conditions for which supervision or approval is required.

A *bandha* stops energy from leaking from the body and can be directed toward different *granthis* to increase circulation of *prana*. The *bandhas* should be done on an empty or digested stomach. They can be done in isolation, with awareness, as part of *asana* (yoga postures) or as one full lock, known as *maha bandha*. The SOSA website (*see p.xxi*) offers a short series of Tantra Yoga classes focused on the *bandhas*, which we'll now explore further.

1. **Mula bandha**: This pierces *brahma granthi* (knots around *Mulhadhara* and *Svadhistana chakras*: pelvis, water functions, lower abdomen, sacrum, lower back, and genitals). It involves contracting different parts of the pelvic floor, along with *kumbak* (breath retention). An important preparatory practice is *ashwini mudra* (the contraction and release of the anal sphincter and urethra, as if you were stopping the flow of pee and then releasing) to gain awareness of the different parts of the pelvic floor. *Mula bandha* is done by inhaling generously to fill the pelvic diaphragm; as you exhale, begin squeezing the perineum, the space between the anus and genitals, along with the rest of the perineal region, inward and upward toward the navel. The lock is held for a few seconds while retaining the breath, and then released slowly, relaxing the muscles with the inhalation.

2. **Uddhiyana bandha**: This pierces *vishnu granthi* (knots around *Manipura* and *Anahata*: stomach, lungs, chest, heart, shoulders, and upper back). This can be done seated with hands on knees, or standing with knees bent and hands resting on the thighs. Inhale and exhale completely in a short, sharp breath. Suck your navel in toward your spine with the suction of the exhale, and pull your navel up toward your heart. As you do this, your chest may lift. To release, gently release the

stomach and slowly inhale. Do not stand up too quickly. Take a few breaths to ground into the earth before moving.

3. **Jalandhara bandha:** This pierces *rudra granthi* (knots around *Vishuddha* and *Ajna*: throat, thyroid, mouth, face, eyes, mind, higher power). Sit comfortably. Inhale until your lungs are about two-thirds full; retain the breath. Drop the chin down and draw it back to your chest (as if making a double chin); lift your chest and sternum back up to the chin. Now, exhale fully and swallow to activate the lock. Relax your shoulders and hold your attention in the throat and center of the forehead, until it feels comfortable to release. Don't wait until you're gasping for air. Trust yourself. To release, gently release your head and slowly inhale. This *bandha* naturally activates in shoulder stand and bridge pose.

4. **Maha bandha:** This is known as the 'great lock,' which is when all three locks are taken together: Start with the *mula bandha*, then move to *uddhiyana bandha*, then lock the throat with *jalandhara bandha* and slowly release to observe the sensations and *shakti* around the body.

Tantra and Trauma

The rational cognitive brain knows how to distinguish between past, present, and future, but for the trauma living in the body, there's only the experience of now, which persists through recurring traumatic sensations. The work of Tantric practice is to allow each person to complete the cycle by working through all layers in the body, to release their *samskaras* and *granthis*, and restore safety of the body, mind and spirit in the present.

Wherever you may be in your own process, however long ago or recent the experiences were, whether they were experienced in your own body or by the generations before you – know there are methods to complete the cycle. You're in the right place to begin to do that, as you read this book and do these practices. Your body and your *shakti* are wise, and as you go on to develop your relationship with them, they'll tell you where the trauma is stored. As you complete the cycles and release the trauma, numbness, fear, or pain from these experiences, you'll create space for more energy, sensation, sensuality, joy, and pleasure to course through your body.

▼ Activities ▼

Shaking and Dynamic Meditations

All mammals shake off trauma, yet for some reason, we humans stopped! A simple yet effective practice is to put on some music and shake your entire body. Music with drums and a fast BPM (beats per minute) is helpful. You can check out the SOSA website for shaking music and a playlist. Incredible dynamic, cathartic meditation music is available at OSHO.com, where this practice originated.

Take 60 minutes to complete the following steps, or halve the times and try for 30 minutes:

1. 10 mins: Breathe chaotically through the nose, without rhythm or pattern, while focusing on the exhalation. Your breath should be fast and hard. Use your body's natural movements to build energy.

2. 10 mins: Explode – let go of everything that needs to be released. Scream, shout, punch pillows, cry, jump, kick, shake, laugh, throw – hold nothing back and keep your whole body moving. If you

don't know what needs releasing, do the movements anyway and see what's released.

3. 10 mins: Jump with your arms raised above your head. Jump up and down, allowing your heels and feet to hammer the ground as you chant the *mantra Hoo, hoo, hoo!* and drive energy into your sex center.

4. 15 mins: Whatever position you're in, stop and freeze – don't move. Be a witness to everything happening within.

5. 15 mins: Celebrate with music: Dance, express, and bring joy and aliveness through your body.

Tantra Yoga

Tantra Yoga is a powerful practice that works on all five *koshas*. It has a deep relation to the energetic body, particularly the *chakra* system. It also works with deities, *mantras*, and *kriyas* to connect to *shakti* as a vital life force for healing, transformation, transmuting trauma, and expanding sensual life force.

You can join SOSA's online Tantra Yoga community from anywhere in the world to integrate these practices and connect with others who are taking the classes at the same time. It's a good place to establish the regularity required to feel the effects of the Tantra Yoga practice and establish your own connection with *shakti each week*.

Tantric Bodywork

Tantric bodywork works with *kundalini shakti* energy to invoke sensual and sexual energy in the body and allow it to guide us toward the blocks, knots, traumas, emotions, and tangles that need addressing and releasing.

The bodyworker will attend to these areas and allow you to release what is stuck there, whether it's physical, emotional, energetic, or mental, to clear the path for shakti, sensuality, and joy to flow. Please note, this is different from Tantric massage or erotic massage, and you should be cautious when finding a bodyworker, making sure you understand the intention of the session.

Bodywork sessions with me can last several hours, or indeed, several sessions in order to allow for the process, integration, and completion of the emotional cycle. You can book these through the SOSA website.

SENSFUL Method with Trauma

The SENSFUL method can be used alone or in a safe space with a friend, therapist, bodyworker, or teacher who can hold space for you.

1. **S – Safety:** Ground the body by connecting to the senses and setting up in a safe and private space.

2. **E – Evoke:** Evoke the sensation through bodywork, cathartic embodiment, journaling or speaking about the experience.

3. **N – Notice:** Notice any sensations coming up for you as you visit these experiences in your mind and body.

4. **S – Sublimate:** Do this by cathartically releasing what you need to about this experience; this might be crying, moving, shouting, screaming, kicking, or shaking, to complete the process.

5. **F – Free:** Express through journaling, speaking about, or sharing what came up for you.

6. **U – Understand:** Understand your experience without judgment of how you feel.

7. **L - Love:** Bring the nervous system back into states of safety through balancing breath, grounding, dance, or affirmation: *I am safe. I am present. I am love. I am sacred.*

Integration

1. Journal about the trauma you've experienced through the lens of your life as an individual.

2. Journal about trauma experienced by any groups you belong to (e.g., race, gender, sexuality, caste, socioeconomic, nationality, etc.)

3. Research the history of your family, country, or culture. Journal on any intergenerational trauma you may have experienced, or that could be experienced.

4. Try any of the suggested activities/practices and journal about your reflections.

Key Takeaways

~ The sensations of trauma can stay stuck in the body and stop us from experiencing the full spectrum of our sensations and sensuality.

~ In Tantric terms, we experience trauma and energetic blockages through the *koshas* (the five layers that comprise the physical, emotional, mental, and spiritual aspects of the self) and the *granthis* (psychic knots in the *koshas*).

~ *Bandhas* are 'locks' that pierce through the *granthis*. A *bandha* keeps energy from leaking from the body and can be directed toward different *granthis* to increase circulation of *prana*.

~ In order to experience the full flow of our *shakti* energy, it's important to close the looping cycle of trauma in the body.

~ Tantra Yoga, psychotherapy, bodywork, and a combination of mind- and body-based activities can be very helpful in closing the cycles of trauma that repeat in the body.

CHAPTER 7

Feeling Fear

Our fears and anxieties are influenced by our experiences, our upbringing, our culture or religion, and our society. In one country, it might be safe to walk down a street alone at night, and in another, it's an unthinkable adventure. In one city, you may feel free to dress as you like, and in another, it may be punishable by law. In one social group, you might feel free to explore your sensuality, and in another, you would be riddled by fear at the thought of it.

Fear and our freedom within it are therefore highly subjective. Anxiety set off by the flame of fear can lead to a wildfire of thoughts that lead us to evaluate a situation through a distorted perspective. The mechanisms we use to keep us safe can be effective, but they can also strengthen the force of fear. If we become afraid of feeling our fear, we build a dam around feeling our sensuality.

A lot of self-help books teach us how to 'overcome' fear and anxiety, but seeing as the force of fear is so strong, this chapter will teach an approach that's a little different – it'll teach us how to harness our fear in service of our *shakti*. Here, we'll give space to fear, not as a frightening foe but as a familiar friend, to learn how to catch its smoke on the winds of our sails and use its charge to open to states of deeper connection, aliveness, and sensuality.

False Evidence Appearing Real

One soft summer's evening, I was hanging out somewhere I thought I was safe and was spiked, without my knowing, with some drops of LSD. Unaware of the spiraling turn I was heading into, I experienced all the defenses my conscious mind had built over the course of my life, to keep me from feeling my deepest fears, come crumbling down.

Simultaneously, I not only saw the depths of fear, but got to experience this in a hospitalized psychosis. I saw, heard, tasted, touched, and felt the darkest night of my soul and its fears as they turned from whispers under the surface into screams that jolted me from the grip of reality into a downward spiral of delusions.

Nothing and no one could be trusted — even the doctors and nurses, even myself. At the time, and for several months, I could feel only anger for the situation and the way it had happened. Now, I'm aware that this was a part of the journey I was meant to take to understand not only those with psychosis — which exists within my family — but the very strong fearful reality existing under the surface of my daily life.

Without my awareness, these fears were driving my thoughts, my decisions, and of course, my reality when I wasn't in a psychotic state. The only difference with someone in psychosis is that those fears draw to the forefront of the mind in delusions that can feel more real than reality itself. But fear, even if we are not in psychosis, feels real to us all — for example, the threat of falling from a high building, or a plane crashing, or a spider biting us. Whether or not the event has actually happened does not relate to whether we experience fear. This is why 'fear' is sometimes turned into an acronym for 'false evidence appearing real.'

If you think of a fear you have right now, you'll feel it in your body as real will you not? So, what then distinguishes fear as psychosis from the fear that lives under the skin of our day-to-day but the quality of discernment? Discernment is the ability to distinguish truth from illusion. Meditation on our fears on the spiritual path is a form of discernment that helps remove the veil of illusion that keeps us contracted, small, unworthy, and scared. It can bring us closer to the truth of our bold, brilliant, courageous spirit, which longs to be seen and known.

Because once you have felt your fears, what else is left to be scared of?

Smoke or Steam?

I once lived in a house in London with some friends and an over-sensitive fire alarm. It detected our morning toast as enough of a threat to go off and wake up the whole street. No matter where we are from, the color of our skin, the size of our house, the language we speak – we all have a fire alarm in our inner default network. Sometimes it goes off because there is a real and serious threat to our lives, but other times it goes off and it's really just the steam from an innocent banana bread baking in the oven.

Our fear sensor has to act very quickly, but can't always discern between a real and a false threat. Our senses only deliver the message and tell us there *could* be something to be alarmed about. It's our job to understand whether it's smoke or steam.

This fear is a deeply rooted paradox of our human instincts that, on one hand, work to keep us alive, but simultaneously block us from fully living, connecting, and expanding on the other side of fear.

When we're young, we might fear the dark or the monster under the bed, until, if we're lucky, an affirming voice tells us, 'Hey, look, there's nothing there,' with a comforting hand on our head, and we learn to fall asleep at night. As we grow older and this comforting voice disappears, our fears often grow into a long list of anxieties, until we no longer jump from one step to another for fear we'll fall, or make that life change we've been thinking about for a number of years for fear we'll fail. So, let's get a good look at this 'block' on the road to expansion: fear.

What Is Fear?

The word *fear* comes from the old English *fær*, which means 'calamity, sudden danger, peril, or sudden attack.' Fear is a built-in system in all humans, designed to protect us from harm, threats, and dangers. Fear is the catalyst of anxiety and can make moments feel uncomfortable or completely overwhelming.

When it dodges us away from traffic, we're grateful it exists. But when we've got a big interview or presentation and it keeps us up all night, it doesn't feel so good. The symptoms of fear fill us with anxiety and flood our bodies with adrenalin.[1] This sets off the screeching fire alarm so we can't focus on anything else, enjoy our senses, or connect to our loved ones in peace. Fear is simply too loud to let us enjoy the sensual world and our sensuous bodies.

In her groundbreaking book *Feel the Fear and Do It Anyway*, Susan Jeffers breaks fear down into three levels.[2] The first level is the surface story, which can be divided into the things that happen to us — aging, illness, retirement, children leaving home, change, death, war, losing a loved one, abuse, accidents, natural disasters, and the things that require action. These include making decisions, leaving or entering relationships, changing careers, making friends, starting a business, improving in a hobby, exercising, having intimate relationships, etc.

The next level of fear involves the inner states of mind, such as fear of rejection, success, failure, vulnerability, helplessness, disapproval, or loss of image. Fear that's felt in one area of life, such as fear of not being successful in our career, can spill into other areas, such as fear of not being successful in our relationships.

The final level of fear is the deepest and the one that keeps us most stuck because it's the biggest fear of all: the belief that we can't handle it. This may come through thoughts such as, *I'm not ready. I can't and I don't know how.* It also includes negotiations and blocks, such as: 'When X happens, I'll do Y. When I've lost enough weight, I'll have better sex. When I'm rich enough, I'll invest my money.' Sound familiar? Whatever 'it' is for you, a big part of our work in this chapter is understanding fear so we can use it to expand our consciousness and experience of life.

Fears About Sensuality

What are some of the most common fears that block our sensuality? These are the ones I've encountered, in myself and the many people who've come through SOSA:

1. **Fear of being seen:** This is about being seen as a sensual being, whether that looks like dancing freely to music, embracing a partner in public, going for a delicious dinner alone, or simply enjoying your senses. It can be influenced by the way

our parents enjoyed their lives; for example, if we saw them do nothing but work, it might raise the fear of being seen enjoying our own lives. It's also about the culture, religion, and society we're raised in, as being sensual or enjoying pleasure and our senses might be confused with being 'sexual,' which can be seen as taboo and make it difficult for us to distinguish sensual from sexual.

2. **Fear of vulnerability:** Sensuality often involves vulnerability because it involves allowing our true self to be known. That means vulnerability with ourselves, which requires breaking the dams we build to keep us from feeling our fears. Then, it might mean sharing what's on the other side of those dams: our fears and our desires, our fantasies and our boundaries. Vulnerability shines a light on deep connection to ourselves and to others.

3. **Fear of rejection:** If we embrace our sensuality or ask for what we want, will we risk not being accepted? We might fear telling someone 'no' because it could hurt their feelings and in turn hurt our own, or we might fear that if we were to bring our whole self – our vulnerable self, our sensual self – it might be 'too much' for the other person to bear. Both hearing rejection and surviving it in small ways can teach us that 'no' is an empowered choice. Practicing saying no to others is also a powerful way to work with rejection. This might look like saying no to going out when you just want to stay in, or asking a waiter for something on the menu that doesn't exist, just to familiarize yourself with the subtle but powerful feelings of rejection and your capacity to handle it.

4. **Fear of the unknown:** This is about stepping outside our comfort zone. We might do this by exploring new sensations or

experiences with ourselves or a partner, by starting that new creative project, by going deeper into pleasure, or by exploring one of the practices in this chapter. Fear of the unknown can be paralyzing, because as much as it keeps us stable and safe, it can also keep us stuck. Whenever you do something new, the sensation of fear will appear. Summon to mind something you used to fear that you can now do without even thinking about it. You can do it!

5. **Fear of intimacy:** This fear can arise from our attachment patterns. For example, according to attachment theory, if our attachment style is 'anxious,' it means we fear being abandoned or alone, which causes us to cling to safety – in our relationships and in what we already know. If our attachment style is avoidant, we fear losing ourselves or our independence, which makes us steer clear of deeply connecting with others. The way we're raised and past traumas can affect our attachment style. Intimacy can be cultivated by sharing thoughts, ideas, emotions, feelings, as well as our senses and spirituality, with ourselves, another, or a higher power.

6. **Fear of recurring trauma:** While trauma is based on what has happened in the past, fear is based on what might happen in the future. It might be based on events that triggered trauma in the past, but the very nature of fear is anticipation, even if we're living under very different circumstances today. As we explored in the previous chapter, its cycle may be repeating as if the experience is happening 'now' in the body, which keeps us from deeper sensuality and connection.

Yogic and Tantric Approaches to Fear

While trauma swings the pendulum in our mind back toward the past, fear and anxiety swing the pendulum from the present and into the future. In yogic philosophy, this swinging pendulum of chit-chat in the mind is called *chitta*, which translates to 'fluctuations.' The first *sutra* (aphorism) of *The Yoga Sutras of Patanjali* defines the purpose of the yoga practice in the line, *Yogas chitta vritti nirodha*, meaning, 'Yoga is the stilling of the fluctuations of the mind.'

Fearful thoughts are a type of *chitta* that makes our internal world fluctuate, and fear is what's known as *maya*, or illusion. Some schools invite us to 'enlighten' or remove ourselves from the material world because it's based on illusion; however, Tantra is particularly interested in fear as a part of the material world because of its high-voltage sensations and the energy it releases in the body. It sees fear as *shakti* with the potential to transform and expand our life.

> *Tantra acknowledges fear as a natural part of human existence and does not seek to rid us of it, to overcome it, or to eliminate it, because this would be dismissing reality as it truly is. Instead, it encourages us to give fear a space to be felt, accepted, and embraced as a part of being human. This acceptance leads to opportunities for expansion.*

As life unfolds around us, Tantra hones our ability to play within it, rather than escape from it. To be both in the divine play of life (known in sanskrit as *leela*) and be able to watch it is what brings us to the *vijnanamaya* and *anandamaya koshas* we explored in the previous chapter.

Four Steps for Moving Through Fear

Now, we can breathe a huge sigh of relief, because if fear is a simple fact of life, there's nothing to get rid of and nothing more to overcome – fear simply exists, like the fire alarm, and we learn how to open doors, fans, and windows in order to navigate it! Fear can be frightening, or it can be fuel for sensual and spiritual growth. Let's explore how we can use it for our growth.

Step 1 – Know your comfort zone

Start with knowing what is within your comfort zone by noticing what is 'normal' to you. You might feel comfortable talking to someone new on a night out but not during the day. You might feel comfortable asking a question online in a seminar but not in person. You might feel comfortable with someone else pleasuring you but be met by fear and icky feelings when giving pleasure to yourself. You can connect with what your fears are by recognizing something you'd like to do or experience but feel unable to.

Step 2 – Feel the fear

We're not necessarily aware of the fears we live with, until we experience them and bring our awareness to them. Think of a fear you have, rational or irrational, present or not. If you close your eyes, breathe, and focus on it, how does it feel? Interocept and notice any sensations. Fear can have a mental, physical, physiological, emotional, energetic, and spiritual response in the body. For some, it might be muscle tension, sweating, a pounding chest, and a heightened state of alertness; for others, it might be a combination of dread, discomfort, and unease. Everything you fear feels real because its sensations are real. This is what makes fear a deeply internal process in which acknowledging our sensations is key. If fear feels overwhelming and overloads you with sensation, there are practices to bring your nervous system back into balance at the end of this chapter. If you're able to feel the fear for 30 seconds one day, 60 seconds the next, 90 seconds the following, and so on, you'll begin to feel more aware of the sensations it brings.

Step 3 – Discern the fear

Since fear will never go away as long as we continue to grow and life draws us into the unknown, the only way to deal with it is to familiarize ourselves with how to move through it. You're not alone – every human shares the feeling of fear; even the ones who seem like they don't have just learned how to navigate it. Once we've felt the sensations in our body, we get to discern: Is this fear a paralysis, or is this fear 'false evidence appearing as real' and potential fuel for growth? Paralysis from fear comes from a feeling of helplessness. Imagine a person scared of heights walking across a bridge held between two mountain peaks; they look down and freeze, unable to go back and unable to move forward. Now, imagine a person who feels the fear and uses it for fuel; they still feel the sensations but use them to navigate to the other side.

As our senses are what create our perception of the world, we can tune in to the sensations delivered to us to gain power over our perceptions. Imagine you're about to present to a hundred people; you feel butterflies in your stomach, your heart rate increases, you feel warmer than normal, and your cheeks flush and turn red. You can feel your breath rise and fall more intensely than normal. In your body, what does this mean? For some of us, it might point to nervousness and fear; for others, it may be called excitement – the sensations are the same, as the body prepares us for the moment, but the perception is different.

To be in touch with our sensual wisdom is to know what our sensations are telling us and make choices accordingly. If we feel flushed, we have the practices at the end of this chapter to 'open the windows' and stop our fire sensor from going off. In our choice to respond to our sensations, we're offered a moment to observe and respond in a way that moves us toward connection with ourselves, people, opportunities, our work, and the world around us. If we react rather than respond to our sensations, we may move in ways that keep us from expanding – by disregarding sensations, taking the opposite action to what they're indicating, or numbing them altogether.

Step 4 – Expand

Rather than running from 0–100, expansion allows us to step a little more out of our comfort zone over time. Over days, months, and years, our efforts accumulate. Each time we take the risk to expand, new sensations will appear, and our *shakti*, our power, and our connection to our sensuous body will grow stronger. Here are two examples:

Fear: what people might think if you were to write a blog

1. Start writing and posting privately for one month.

2. The next month, make the blog public so strangers can see it.

3. The next month, send it to five people you know.

4. The next month, send it to 10 more people you know.

5. The next month, post it on your social media.

Fear: expressing your desires to your partner

1. Start by writing your desires down in a journal.

2. Read them each day for a week, so you become familiar with how they feel as you say them.

3. The following week, say them out loud every day in front of the mirror.

4. The following week, ask a friend to practice expressing and talking about it.

5. The following week, ask your partner if you can talk to them about your desires.

Think about something you fear now and use this five-step incremental process for expansion over the next five weeks. To help you on your way, there's a Tantric goddess for overcoming fear and embracing transformation. Let's meet her here.

Goddess Kali

Kali Ma translates to 'the mother goddess of darkness.' She represents time, transformation, endings, and beginnings. She is the slayer of fears that lead us away from knowing our true, sacred, divine nature. Her energy involves us in a cycle that stimulates our growth. Kali represents the 'audacious fierceness that has historically been denied both to the divine feminine in all beings and to individual women.'[3] She helps us stand up for ourselves, discover our wild side, harness our unique power, and embrace our sexuality.

Knowing this goddess will help us to see the darkness and fears inside ourselves so that we may acknowledge our potential. As one of the most common human fears is death, Kali is known for living in the cremation grounds, where Tantric practice began. In some schools, advanced practitioners meditated on the corpse of someone who had just died, to come face to face with the fear of death and sublimate its energy for spiritual evolution.

Kali helps us overcome the masks we've built through self-limiting beliefs, patterns, fears, or attachments that stop us from moving forward. The death of these things can create fertile ground for transformation and new beginnings.

According to psychology, we rely on our birth parents or mothers to provide a 'good object,' or a space for us to process the difficult aspects of living as we grow. Kali Ma provides us an opportunity to contact and create our own internal mother, who cares for us and guides us to be courageous in understanding the things we fear — be that ending a relationship, looking at our trauma, embracing our sensuality, or making a career change.

Kali appears in the Atharvaveda, a collection of hymns and mantras published between 1200 BCE and 1000 BCE. Later, around 600 BCE, she is described in the Devi Mahatmyam with the goddess Durga on the battlefield. In other texts, such as the Linga Purana and the Vamana Purana (1100–500 CE), she is described alongside her counterpart, Shiva. Over time, her myths have morphed, but her underlying untamable presence remains.

Let's explore a myth of the goddess Kali from the Linga Purana.

Kali's Rage

A demon name Daruka is wreaking havoc on earth. Shiva approaches his wife, Parvati, to destroy the great demon. Knowing their powers will be better in union, Parvati enters Shiva's body and finds poison in Shiva's throat. From this poison, she transforms. Her skin grows darker and darker, and her presence larger and larger.

Soon, the color of her skin deepens to the color of the darkest night sky. She becomes larger and more ferocious, as she transforms into Kali Ma. Kali is intoxicated by the battle, and her rage becomes uncontrollable. She is ready to destroy anything that enters her path.

As Kali begins drinking the blood of her enemies, Shiva realizes he is no longer in the presence of his beloved Parvati. The more anyone tries to control Kali, the angrier she becomes. Shiva, knowing Kali can destroy the Earth, needs to figure out how to contain this ever-expanding energy. And so, the powerful god of death and destruction lies on the ground, still as a corpse.

As Shiva takes his corpse pose, *savasana*, lying inert on the ground, Kali steps on him. Shiva represents consciousness, which gives a space for Kali's rage, fear, and vengeance to be witnessed, seen, and heard. This expanding and overwhelming energy is contained and understood. Together, with consciousness (Shiva) and power (Kali), they restore the world to peace.

This story reminds us that we're all capable of feeling our emotions, even the ones that may feel repressed in society, when we're able to hold space for them with consciousness.

Connecting with Kali
I invite you to develop a relationship with this divine mother goddess who leads us through fear toward transformation.

1. Visualize her image (you can also find this on the SOSA website, *see p.xxi*) or meditate on her visual form or *yantra*, and see what arises.

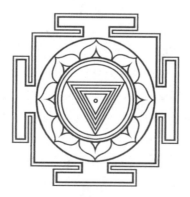

Kali yantra

2. You may wish to listen to a Kali *mantra* when you feel your fear, or to chant one. *Om krim kalikaye namahah* is a powerful invocation that roughly translates to 'I bow to you, Kali.'

3. Try *Kali asana* in your Tantra Yoga practice. Stand with feet wide and sink into your knees or into a deep squat with each pulse. With bent elbows, raise your arms straight out. As you sink into your knees swiftly, shout 'Ahhh,' and stick out your tongue. If you wish, you can hold this posture statically and transmute this energy into power to combat your fears. Notice what you feel afterward.

4. Meditate on the myth of Kali and what it means to you.

5. Close your eyes and imagine Kali Ma before you. Ask her to tell you about how she manifests. You might ask: 'Who are you for me? What can you teach me? Where are you suppressed in me? How can I express you through my life?' Journal any insights you receive.

6. To get to know Kali more deeply, join the Mahavidya Goddesses Tantra Yoga course through SOSA.

▼ Activities ▼

Face Fear in the Moment with Alternate Nostril Breathing

This practice is *anulom vilom*, or a form of alternate nostril breathing, during which you use your fingers and thumb to alternate between opening and closing your nostrils. This breath helps regulate the nervous system from overwhelm and bring you back to a state of balance, so you can make a more informed decision about the fear or anxiety that may be arising.

The following steps are for a right-handed person. If you are left-handed, use the index and middle fingers to close the right nostril first (Step 4) and the thumb to close the left (Step 5).

1. Sit or stand comfortably, and close your eyes.

2. Start by taking a deep breath in and exhaling out.

3. Close the right nostril with your thumb.

4. Slowly inhale, sipping the air through the left nostril (you can do this for a count of 4–20 seconds, increasing as you practice over time).

5. Close your left nostril with your index and middle fingers, and slowly exhale for the same amount of time through the right nostril.

6. Slowly inhale through the right nostril and then close it with your thumb as you slowly exhale through the left nostril.

Repeat this for as long as you need to bring your body back into a state of balance.

Always finish with the left nostril open.

The Five Senses Grounding Technique

If panic, anxiety, or fear catches you in the moment, using the five senses is an incredible way to ground your thoughts and calm your nervous system.

1. **Sight:** Notice and name colors or objects you see around you.

2. **Sound:** Notice and name sounds you hear.

3. **Smell:** Notice and name scents you smell.

4. **Taste:** Notice and name tastes in your mouth.

5. **Touch:** Notice where you can feel your body touching the earth, or bring your hand to touch a part of your body and notice the sensations there.

Slow Exposure Therapy

Exposure therapy is a treatment that helps people confront their fears. While avoidance might help us in the short-term, long-term avoidance will expand the sensations of fear within us. A program of exposure therapy can be worked out with a therapist to help break patterns of avoidance and fear. A safe environment is created in which to expose the individual slowly to anything that's avoided and feared; these might include activities, situations, or environments. This is particularly helpful for phobias, panic disorders, obsessive compulsive disorder (OCD), post-traumatic stress disorder (PTSD), anxiety disorder, and social anxiety disorder.[4]

Expansion and Contraction Meditation

Spanda is a Tantric concept that describes the pulsation of consciousness through all phenomena. It is the subtle contraction and expansion in all things. The breath comes in and expands our lungs, then the breath goes out and voids our lungs. Our eyes blink open and shut. The lotus closes in the day and opens in the night. You get the idea.

The rhythm of music and even our heart is experienced through both vibration and silence. Think of it as the pulse of the *shakti* that flows through me, you, and all things in nature. On your pathway to sensuality, you may feel this contraction through shame, trauma, fear, or anxiety. Invite it to be there by moving into the *vijnanamaya kosha* (see p.136) to witness it. Watch it knock on the door, and if you can, get up to do the practice, walk to therapy, or step on your mat, anyway.

On the other side of fear, resistance, and contraction, you'll create space for allowing your sensual life force to flow, and see the expression of sensual expansion trickle from *kosha* to *kosha*. Through a series of contractions and expansions, you'll build a path toward *anandamaya*, the bliss body, and build the sensual wisdom that allows you to access it.

SENSFUL Meditation for Fear

1. **S - Safety:** Sit somewhere comfortable and close your eyes. Ground and notice the sensations in your body as you arrive, with a few deep breaths. Feel the expansion of your ribs, lungs, and heart space as you inhale. Notice the contraction of your body as you exhale. Meditate on this as a manifestation of the *spanda* that pulses through the universe and within.

2. **E – Evoke:** Bring forth one of your fears and meditate on what it looks, sounds, and feels like in your body

3. **N – Notice:** Take note of where you feel the sensations of contraction in your body. Don't try to fight, change, or ground yourself. Say to yourself, 'I feel my heart pounding. I feel my palms sweating,' until you come to notice everything that's happening within. Do this for 30 seconds and gradually increase the duration each time you do the meditation.

4. **S – Sublimate:** Soothe yourself by breathing deeply, exhaling generously, grounding your body into the earth, and noticing your senses and how you can both experience your fear and be safe in your body. If the charge is high in the body, shake for a few minutes or do a grounding meditation.

5. **F – Free:** Ask yourself with discernment: Is this *maya* (illusion/false evidence appearing real)? Meditate on what's on the other side of fear. Share the sensations arising in your body, through journaling or speaking.

6. **U - Understand:** Where might this fear come from? What has encouraged this fear to strengthen over the course of your life? What would the other side of this fear look like?

7. **L - Love:** Affirm to yourself: *I am love. I am shakti. I am powerful and have what I need to face my fears.* Arrive back in your seat by taking a few breaths. Journal about what came up for you, including action steps to bring you through the fear to the other side. Then, take the action!

Integration

1. Write down any fears you used to have in the past but which no longer exist – remind yourself, 'I can do it!'

2. Write down any fears you have now that you avoid. Notice where you feel them in your body.

3. How do you experience Kali energy (the power to transform and move through fear) in your life? What is in your shadow that could be brought forth with Kali?

4. Try out one of the practices in this chapter and reflect on what came up for you.

Key Takeaways

~ Fear is an inner fire alarm that cannot be removed but can be befriended.

~ There are many fears associated with sensuality: fear of being seen, fear of vulnerability, fear of rejection, fear of the unknown, fear of intimacy, and fear of recurring trauma.

~ Fearful thoughts are a type of *chitta*, or 'fluctuation,' inside our internal world, and fear is what's known as *maya*, or illusion. Tantra is interested in fear because of its intense energy, which can be channeled as transformative *shakti* and used to expand.

~ There are four important steps for moving through fear: stepping out of your comfort zone, feeling the fear, discerning the fear, and expanding.

~ Kali Ma is a powerful Tantric goddess who represents time, transformation, endings, and beginnings. Her intense energy has the ability to stimulate our growth and shake the foundations of our illusions so we can move beyond our fears into expansion.

CHAPTER 8

Feeling Stress

The 21st century is an incredible period of time to live in. The technology boom has taken us to the farthest planets and into the depths of the ocean. Social media has connected us across the globe. Laptops and mobile devices mean we can work from beachfront bars or while wearing messy buns in our living rooms. However, the tools that connect us with each other can be the same ones that disconnect us from our bodies, sensations, and relationships. With the world at our fingertips, we're left with less and less time to simply *be*. We're presented with more and more to do, and as such, human beings have become human doings.

The more we experience society's framework, *action + energy = reward*, the more our neural pathways learn to produce and place our value on what we do rather than who we are. Stress becomes our resting state. When we apply this equation to sensuality, we can feel disappointed, frustrated, or confused when the same formula doesn't work and we're left feeling disconnected and wondering what to do.

Our sensuality isn't something we can put on speed dial or access with the click of a button. Sensuality isn't a goal — it's a state of being, with its own intelligence, which has evolved and developed over many millennia. In this chapter, we'll unpack this together and explore practices that lead us out of sensuality as transient bursts of stress and into sensuality as waves of deep and lasting pleasure.

Hitchhiking through Resistance

Straight from law school, with a bunch of questions still in my heart and a body full of stress, I went on a journey to sit with monks, guides, and gurus around the world, a journey I am still on to date. Every time I closed my eyes and tried to imitate the people around me, sitting in what looked like silent bliss, my mind would spark up in a cacophony of to-do lists, intrusive thoughts, and mental clutter. No matter how much I tried, my mind would simply not rest. My body was full of tension, aches, and pains; this vicious cycle led to inner whispers: 'You're not made to meditate.'

One summer in 2016, I stayed in a Buddhist community in Eastern Thailand that changed my life, perhaps for the very reason I'm about to share with you. You could only access the community through a series of cross-country night buses and by hitchhiking along uncertain paths and fields. The journey to the community was an initiation in and of itself.

The community was started by a former Buddhist monk who, through his loving and playful ways, created a place like nothing I had never experienced before. We woke and meditated together, practiced yoga together, cooked together, ate together, cleaned together, shared our joys and worries, and rested our heads on the earth, under a tarpaulin where we fell asleep together, as electric fireflies glowed in the dark around us. It was in this community where I first felt empowered to share my story publicly. It was this monk who first gave me the insight that it was my path to study and teach yoga.

In the practices where I just couldn't shake the stress, tension and thoughts from my mind and body, he shared with us in his daily *satsang* (spiritual discourse) an incredible insight for the resistance I was feeling toward meditating, practicing yoga, or doing anything that brought me into my body or heart. He said, 'The mind will always battle against the activities which will weaken its power. This is because the very job of the mind is to keep us safe, to minimize use of energy for its own maximum output and keep us in the comfort of what we know, even if all we know is stress, fear, shame. Expanding beyond what we know takes energy, and when the mind doesn't like this, it offers us resistance: *Meditation isn't for you; you can't do that yoga pose; this practice is boring.*'

Hearing the mind and its thoughts of resistance can be powerful, for it's where we step into *vijnanamaya kosha* and are able to see it as separate from our true self. I realized I had spent many years, as most of us reading this will have, in education that trained my mind, and made it much stronger than the will of my body, intuition, or spirit. Now, the path is to pour the same devotion we give to our mental studies into training our heart, senses, and body, which carries a wellspring of untapped and limitless wisdom.

What Is Stress?

Stress comes from the old French *estresse*, meaning 'narrowness' or 'oppression.' It's based on the Latin *strictia*, meaning 'drawn tight, compressed, or drawn together.' This is fitting, as the sensations of stress can often feel like a tightness or compression in the body.

Stress is often used to describe a myriad events: from exams at school to deadlines at work, from picking up the kids between meetings to getting all the housework and life admin done on the weekends. Stress, as we all know, appears in direct response to what's happening in the outside world; it can become a mirror of your tasks, your to-do list, and what you feel is expected of you.

In order to meet these demands, your body will switch from the parasympathetic nervous system, also known as the 'rest and digest' system, to the sympathetic nervous system, which releases cortisol, the stress hormone, and glucose in the bloodstream to give us the energy to do what we need to do. This will make the organs and muscles work harder to meet the demands of the task at hand, causing our senses to sharpen. If you're setting off on a run, the release of energy will be different from what occurs if you're being chased by a lion. Sometimes, that lion might come in the form of a deadline for work or a series of long and grueling days without rest.

When the charge and energy of stress is high in the body, and not in direct proportion with the amount we actually need to complete our to-do list, we might find the holds an excess charge – meaning we have difficulty falling asleep, relaxing, engaging fully in our senses, or enjoying our sensuality. This is what makes stress the final block we explore in this chapter.

Over time, if stress does not find a channel to release or transmute, it begins to be held unconsciously in the body, through clenched jaws and tight muscles, racing hearts and a general feeling of discomfort and dis-ease. If the equation of stress goes unbalanced without regulation or outlet, this can lead to burnout. It can also weaken our immunity and become a

chronic state. Life as we know it becomes a lot less
enjoyable, and, therefore, a lot less sensual.

This is why ancient systems such as Ayurveda, Yoga, and Tantra are based on teaching the body, time and again, how to understand its different energies, so that we can make use of healthy stress and disperse excess energy. We'll look at some of these techniques later in this chapter.

Stress and Sensuality

Stress has a direct relationship to our sensuality. The Dual Control Model of Sexual Response,[1] developed in the 1990s by Erick Janssen and John Bancroft, explores what it takes to get to sexual arousal, and how external stimuli can lead to sexual responsiveness.

The model shares that the central nervous system is made up of accelerators and brakes. Your sympathetic nervous system (activated in a stress state) is related to inhibitory processes that block arousal; your parasympathetic nervous system ('rest and digest' state) is represented by the excitatory processes that open arousal through the senses.

In other words, when we are stressed, our body hits the brakes on sensuality, sexuality, and arousal; when the body is relaxed, it hits the accelerator. Janssen and Bancroft call the accelerator the Sexual Excitation System and the brakes the Sexual Inhibition System.

▼ **Accelerator:** This gathers all the sex-related stimuli from our environment and thoughts, and through our senses. It sends a signal to the body, mind, and genitals to turn on. It operates in the unconscious, and we won't often realize it's working until we feel turned on.

- ▼ **Brake 1:** This gathers all of our senses to look out for potential threats. If it gauges threats, it sends a signal to our sexual response to turn off, so we can do what we need to manage that stress.

- ▼ **Brake 2:** This gathers all our senses, but it hits arousal a little bit harder, like a hand brake, and is associated with fear of performance failure. For example, this can manifest in the fear of not being wet enough, hard enough, or beautiful enough, or in failing to reach orgasm.

Many problems we face with our sensuality can be solved by understanding the balance of brakes and accelerators. If you're not getting turned on, sex educator Emily Nagoski shares, 'there's not enough stimulation to the accelerator and too much stimulation for the brakes.' She shares how most people who struggle with desire, sex, and sensuality often think to look at the accelerator.[2]

When we apply this to sensuality, we might hear ourselves say, 'There aren't enough candles, not enough romance, not enough time, not enough XYZ,' but what we really need to do is take our foot off the brakes, reducing perceptions of threat and balancing levels of stress so there's enough to get around our day, but not so much that it blocks access to our sensual stimuli to evoke joy, pleasure, and aliveness.

Sensuality, Stress, and Stimuli

The bridge between arousal and non-arousal is the stimuli from our senses. This arousal is different to sex. Remember, sex is sensual but sensuality isn't just sex.

Sensuality is the way we interact with the world through our senses — how aroused we are with life. Sensual energy can be used to bring more joy, aliveness, creativity, and connection to life when it is channeled as a vital force. The stimuli from our senses will either press the brakes or hit the accelerator on our sexual energy, which we can relate to *kundalini shakti*. This creates inhibition or excitation, and directly reflects the way stress blocks our sensual responses.

Here, we'll look at three stimuli that create stress when it comes to sensuality.

1. **Porn:** In this era, many people's first stroke of sexual energy comes from porn. Today, porn videos make up a third of online traffic globally. In 2018, a study found that porn sites have more traffic than most major news organizations. With porn's ease of access and affordability, many of us learn the ropes of sex and sensuality from what we see. Porn itself isn't a bad thing; in fact, conscious porn, which pays its performers well and ensures that experiences are sensual and consensual, does exist. However, most porn creates unrealistic expectations of the time it truly takes for the body to open. It creates stress and the pressure to become aroused as quickly as the two-minute clip. The visual stimulus of porn does a great job of making goal-oriented sex the primary intimate connection. Unfortunately, the bridge of sensuality usually gets edited out of the frame.

2. **Hedonism and Sexualization:** Many people fear that enjoying the sensual world will mark them as overly sexual or hedonistic. There's a fear that simply enjoying one's senses, sensations, and body could be interpreted as a sexual invitation, or that we may be perceived as promiscuous —

giving rise to shame and causing us to withdraw into the shadows. Much of this comes from the sensual script we grew up with from our culture, family, and society, and also the dangers, catcalls, whistles, and uninvited attention we've received. This creates more reason for us to hit the brakes and perceive our *kundalini shakti* energy as a threat. Yet many of the people I have met and shared practices with have a deep desire to be seen expressing their true, authentic, sensual selves, whether that's through movement, or the way they dress or interact with the world around them. Our work is to reclaim our *kundalini shakti* and sensual expression by looking at the sensual script within, healing from these experiences, and rewiring our minds and bodies to make space for enjoying the world through our senses.

3. **Performance:** The pressure of performance causes us to act as if our sensuality must be expressed solely for another. A participant in a workshop shared how in most underwear shops, outfits and lingerie we're encouraged to wear for a partner are often at the front, but the tools for sexual energy that we use to pleasure ourselves are locked away in a box at the back. The media often rewards externalized sensuality when it meets the needs of consumerism, meaning sensuality gets further externalized and commodified. But sensuality is a way to connect to the world within through our senses, to expand our vital life force, to harness our creativity, and to know our spirit. If more of us can be empowered to live sensually — with the knowledge that it isn't wrong, selfish, or only used in pursuit of external validation — we'll open the door for others to feel sensually empowered.

In the next parts of this chapter, we'll look at how we can transition to feeling a deeper sensuality. Before we get there, something to note is that stress, much like all of the other blocks we have explored in this book, is not always the devil it's made out to be.

For example, stress is required to keep the body standing; without a certain amount of stress, our bones, muscles, and ligaments would melt into a puddle of human parts the moment we took a step. Stress is also the activating agent that prepares us for important moments that require the full and focused attention of our senses.

Many mindfulness or work-based mental-health exercises are about 'reducing stress' and making us 'stress-free.' But the point isn't to demonize or further repress stress. Just as we've learned to navigate shame, trauma, and fear, we'll learn how to ride the waves of stress and honor its presence as a natural part of life.

Stress vs. Rest in Self-Pleasure

In another workshop on sensuality and sex, one participant at the end asked me, 'But isn't every orgasm just a release of stress?' I smiled, as I knew that one well: the orgasm that's just a big sneeze in the pelvis, followed by a lapse of energy, which is comforting enough to blow the stress out and fall asleep afterwards.

A 'stress orgasm' absolutely does the trick, but there's another way to experience deeper sensuality, intimacy, and connection – to draw that energy inward.

'Rest orgasms' are less about chasing a goal and imploding the stress, and more about building peaks and troughs where pleasure rises, falls, and builds, as well as works through the body to heal.

In the Tantra Yoga community at SOSA, our classes teach the body to withstand a certain amount of stress from the postures; this is contrasted with moments of stillness and rest in which you observe the sensations and *shakti* in your body. This teaches the body how, even off the mat, it can switch from stress to rest in a moment. In self-pleasure, you can explore this through a practice known as edging, which builds a certain amount of stress in the body — for example, while self-pleasuring — but contrasts with moments of stillness and rest.

The moments of rest are when sensations and sensuality build. This allows stress to rise and fall. It removes the goal-oriented focus and allows us to experiences waves of *shakti* and sensual pleasure that course through the body inward, rather than expelling through the body outward.

Where this sensual energy courses through the body, it'll find obstacles that are in its way — such as tension; pain; stress; and physical, energetic, or emotional blocks — and use that wave of energy to release and shift those obstacles. This is how sensual energy becomes a healing practice for self-vitalization!

The Goddess of Rest

Rest is revolutionary because society doesn't reward it. But your body and your sensuality do. Rest is central to sensuality, because it is in the stillness that we feel *shakti*; take the foot off the brakes; and allow our senses to draw in stimuli that allow joy, pleasure, creativity, and arousal to accelerate.

You are not missing out when you tune in. The same way we might turn the knob of an old radio to get to the right station, we tune in to the frequency of our sacred messengers, which are being sent out across the magnificent landscape of our body. This leads us to another type of yoga that doesn't require doing anything and welcomes us back to being.

Yoga nidra is sometimes called a form of yogic sleep, but it isn't the sleep we take every night into the unconscious; instead, it's a form of sleep that brings us deep consciousness, rest, refreshment, insight, and revitalization. It doesn't require meditating with a straight and stiff spine, but rather, lying down in comfort and ease. It's less about getting and more about receiving.

Nidra Devi is also a goddess form of *shakti*, the divine power of sleep that no body can resist. She appears in the Rig Veda in hymns and myths, as the bestower of spiritual power who informs us that even gods and goddesses require rest and sleep.[3] *Yoga nidra* is, simply put, the power of conscious rest; it uses special relaxation exercises, guided imagery, and the breath to bring us into a relaxed, receptive, and conscious state.

In her book on *yoga nidra*, Julie Lusk talks about it as a direct tool for reducing stress and breaks the process into three stages:[4]

1. **First stage:** The mind will calm and the body will begin to feel relaxed and heavy.

2. **Second stage:** The heaviness in the body lifts, and a lighter feeling arises.

3. **Third stage:** This is a state between waking and sleep, in which you float in and out of a dreamlike consciousness.

When first practicing *yoga nidra*, you may find you drift off, which is perfectly welcome, as that's what *shakti* needs to do in the body — but with time, you may be able to stay aware of a certain timeless spaciousness while your body and mind are resting. Even

10–20 minutes is sufficient to feel the regeneration of mind, body, and spirit. If you're able to rest with deep and conscious awareness for an undisclosed period of time – for example, after a yoga class – without a timer, chime, or teacher to wake you up again, you can journey into dimensions of the conscious, subconscious, and unconscious mind. You can ride the waves as you come in and out with your breath, visions, and experience.

This is the power that teaches our minds and bodies to connect with deeper intuition, healing, and sensuality – not through stress and goal-driven explosions, but through rest and receiving. You'll find a guided *yoga nidra* practice on the SOSA website.

Conscious Sensuality

To grow deeper in our sensuality, we need to grow more conscious of it. Shiva, whom we met in the myth of Kali in the last chapter, is the cosmic counterpart of Shakti in philosophy and mythology. Like Shakti, Shiva is both a deity and a universal force.

While *shakti* is matter and the manifest world, *shiva* is consciousness and the unmanifest. Without matter, there is nothing to be conscious of – and without consciousness, matter doesn't exist. Shiva and Shakti as deities are presented as cosmic lovers through the ages who long to be with each other.

If *shakti* is our sensuality, all our sensations, and our senses, then *shiva* is our conscious awareness of them. Sometimes, *shiva* is confused in the Western world as the 'divine masculine' and is associated with doing, action-taking, and authoritative energy. But just as we have learned with *shakti*, a concept that goes beyond the 'divine feminine,' *shiva* expands beyond gender associations and social definitions of feminine or masculine. *Shiva* is simply consciousness. We all have *shakti* and *shiva* energy within us.

Rest assured that embarking on the path to conscious sensuality doesn't mean meditating in a cave for years to deepen consciousness. It means moving into a state of awareness, whether in moments of conscious rest, as we explored previously, or being present while you, eat, see, smell, listen, and touch. These meditations of becoming more conscious of the senses are sometimes called *feeding the goddess*.

One way to feed the goddess is at your altar space, as we explored in Chapter 1, by making offerings that evoke each of the senses. Another way of feeding the goddess is bringing deeper consciousness to the way we interact with our senses in our daily life. This is how *shiva* and *shakti* unite within us. When we move fast and indulge in the senses without awareness, we are said to starve *shiva*, and when we live life without the senses and our sensuality, we are said to starve *shakti*!

Like the representations of the deities, these energies long to know each other and dance with fulfillment in your heart. On the following pages you'll learn a practice for bringing more shiva consciousness to the senses through the Journey of the Senses, which you can share with a friend or partner. But first, let's meet Shiva.

Meeting Shiva

Shiva means 'auspicious one.' In mythology, he is an ascetic god living in the Himalayas, and is the creator of Yoga, Tantra, and dance.

He wears a tiger skin around his waist, and his skin is smothered in white ash, with his hair in matted dreadlocks coiled at the top of his head. His neck is blue, as he is capable of drinking even the deadliest of poisons to protect his devotees. The center of his forehead is anointed with a third eye, representing his position as the *adi yogi*, or first yogi, and helping him to distinguish truth from illusion, known as *maya*.

He wears a crescent moon in his hair, and just as the moon waxes and wanes, he tunes in to the rhythm of the cosmos. In one hand he holds a *dhamaru*, a drum, as he dances to the beat of endings and beginnings. He is known as Nataraja, the King of Dance, and his dance is known as the *Tandava* (Sanskrit for 'frantic dancing'). He is responsible for endings and destruction and helps us, along with his *shakti* – Parvati, Kali, Durga – to transform.

▼ Activities ▼

Nadi Shodana

This practice is similar to the alternate nostril breathing (*anulom villom*) we explored in the last chapter; however, it involves holding the breath in a pause between switching the nostrils after the inhale, and holding the breath in a pause at the end of the exhale. It can be helpful to have a count - for example, four counts per inhale and exhale, and four counts for the retention of the breath - that you increase over time. Sometimes, people call this 'box breath' and visualize drawing a box in their mind, or they open their eyes and trace the lines of a window or anything square-shaped, in time with the breath. The pause is where we connect to *shiva* consciousness – it helps break the patterns of stress and return the body to its resting state.

Activity: Sense-Infused Dining

Cook and eat a beautiful meal with all of your senses, which can help you slow down and just be. Try to do this alone, or if with others, in silence to heighten all of the senses. You could also make this a daily ritual with your morning tea or coffee.

1. See: See the colors as you cook and as you eat.

2. Touch: Feel the textures of each ingredient with your hands and mouth.

3. Hear: Listen to the sounds of the food being chopped, cooked, and crunched as you eat.

4. Smell: Smell the scents of each individual ingredient coming together before you eat.

5. Taste: Close your eyes and experience the different flavors and notes – sweet, salty, sour, bitter, and umami (meaty/savory).

Harnessing Sensual Energy Through Self-Pleasure

This edging practice is done through solo self-pleasure or with a partner. You bring yourself to arousal through relaxing the body, connecting to the senses, massaging your body, and then self-pleasuring.

Using a scale of 0 to 10, we designate 0 as not aroused and 10 as orgasm. Bring yourself to a 7, then stop and pause, allowing the stress/tension to relax as you observe the sensations and breathe with awareness.

When the 7 has come back down to a 2 or 3, begin to build it up again to 7; stop and allow the sensual energy to expand through your breath, observing and noticing the sensations. Continue to do this as many times as you like, to build waves of pleasure rather than a peak explosion.

In the moments of pause, you may also direct the energy with your attention to areas in your body you feel would benefit from the fresh *shakti* energy; this could be somewhere you'd like to heal or receive strength/power. At first, it may be difficult to stop, but it'll come with practice!

Journey to the Senses

This is a great way to explore the meditative play of the senses. SOSA and this practice were featured in the Louis Theroux Production documentary *Sex Actually*, in the third episode of the first season. We have a version of this practice online, which can be done as a guided Tantric date night with a partner. You can also do the steps at home.

1. Create a beautiful, sacred temple space with candles, incense, and beauty.

2. Have a comfortable space to lie down, with plenty of space to move around, using mats, pillows, and blankets.

3. Prepare a tray of the senses, which will include:

    ▼ Smell: Prepare a few scents, using essential oils directly on your skin or cotton wool on which to dab the oils, as well as fresh herbs.

    ▼ Taste: Include a few pieces of cut juicy fruit, a few pieces of lemon or lime, and a few pieces of chocolate, for three different tastes.

    ▼ Sound: Prepare a beautiful piece of music with deep meaning for you; allow one song for each person in this exercise, or choose spontaneously in the moment.

    ▼ Touch: Prepare a few different textures, like a silk scarf and feather, or something with more texture. You can also use different types of touch.

    ▼ Sight: Prepare a blindfold for the person receiving.

4. Arrive into the space by connecting through dance, conversation, or eye gazing. Then, place the blindfold on the person receiving and guide them to lie down with their blindfold on and relax each part of their body.

5. Slowly proceed in the order of the senses (smell, taste, sound, touch). Tantalize, tease, and evoke each sense as you go. The person receiving is deprived of the sense of sight, so they are trusting you to look after them. All of their senses will be heightened.

6. If possible, limit communication to the senses. The giver must pay attention to how the person receiving is moving their body. If you as the giver sense they're feeling delight or pleasure, invite them to breathe into their heart space. Use the mantra, 'Divine one, breathe into the heart of the lotus,' which can transmute and expand the sensation across their body.

7. The final sense is sight; bring the person up to a seat and take off their blindfold. You'll witness each other's presence with your sight and deep appreciation.

8. Complete, and swap positions for receiver and giver. There's no goal to move into anything. This is a meditation on the senses in the present.

9. Complete and integrate the practices by sharing your experiences. Reflect on how it was to trust your partner, which senses brought delight, and how you felt during the journey.

▲▲▲

Integration

1. How does stress feel in your body?

2. Are you feeling any stress right now? What demands is this charge of stress trying to meet?

3. Accelerators and brakes: How do you take your foot off the brake or show stress a channel to leave the body? (This could be anything that relaxes you!) Also, what is an accelerator for you? This is something that brings arousal from the senses.

4. Try one of the practices in this chapter and reflect on what you find.

KEY TAKEAWAYS

~ Stress is a direct response to the demands of life. When its charge in the body is disproportionate or not dispersed, it affects sensuality.

~ The Dual Control Method of Sexual Response helps us understand how stress can impact our experiences of sensuality and sexuality through accelerators and brakes.

~ Over time, if stress does not find a channel to release or transmute, it's held unconsciously in the body, through a general feeling of discomfort and dis-ease.

~ Three stimuli that create stress when it comes to sensuality are porn, hedonism and sexualization, and performance.

~ A stress orgasm can release orgasmic energy, but we can experience more sensuality, intimacy, and connection when we draw that energy inward. We can do this through a practice like edging, which allows orgasmic energy to course through the body to nourish our bodies instead of expelling it outward and depleting ourselves.

~ *Yoga nidra* is a form of yogic sleep that brings us deep consciousness, rest, refreshment, and revitalization to combat stress.

~ In exploring conscious sensuality, we can play with feeling the energies of *shakti* (including our senses) and *shiva* (including our awareness) in the body.

PART III

Your Sensual
Rebirth

In Part II, we rafted down the river of sensuality to meet the rocks that block our access to it. Now that we've worked through the blocks, it's time to see what else sensuality can provide us with – it's time for our sensual rebirth.

In this part of the book, you'll discover that your sensual energy doesn't need to be something that is outsourced primarily for the enjoyment of others. With this knowledge, you'll move into the phase of sensual wisdom, which reveals how your sensuality can be pulled inward for your own nourishment, healing, creativity, manifestation, expression, and relationships.

CHAPTER 9

Meeting the
Manifester Within

A s we'll explore in this chapter, when you manifest, you don't just attract what you want to have; you attract who you become. Through this collaboration between mind, sensuality, and spirit, manifestation can also bring us into a deeper connection with ourselves and the universe — because each expression of manifestation is an expression of our most authentic desires combined with the power and belief that we're worthy of them. This becomes a conversation between the forces that spin the wheels of our inner cosmos, whose sacred messengers communicate through sensations, and those of the *parashakti*, the great cosmic forces that spin the planets.

This is a powerful system engineered to transform what you think into what you have and who you are. Manifestation is the ability to move an energy into an action and bring the unmanifest into the manifest. As you have moved through this book and the practices to unlock and expand your sensuality, you've also unlocked within you the power of manifestation to bring your dreams and aspirations into fruition. You'll be pleased to know it's a much simpler process to manifest when you're connected to your sensuality, because it's a practice that involves engaging all of your senses. In this chapter, you'll learn how.

Mini Manifester

Around the age of seven, I got home from school, put my bag down, and got ready to catch up on my favorite TV programs. There were some cartoons I enjoyed, but every day at five, I watched *Blue Peter*, a program for the kids who grew up with static televisions and its few but wonderful channels.

I loved this show, which encompassed adventure, creativity, information, and play. One day, they had a section that followed the lives of athletes. I recall exactly where I stood in the living room, fidgeting and moving, unable to sit still.

They interviewed an Olympic sprinter who was training for a race and asked what he did to prepare. To my surprise, it wasn't just running. The athlete shared that when he set his foot on the starting blocks and waited for the signal to run, he spent those moments with his eyes closed, imagining he had won the race. He wouldn't just see it in his mind's eye. He would feel himself passing the line through the soles of his feet. He would hear the stadium erupt into cheers. Most importantly, he imagined the sensation he would feel and the euphoria in his body at that precise moment. He said this was the final thing, after all his training, that really set him up to win his race.

I felt like I was hearing the secrets of a magician pulling a rabbit from a hat. Keen to explore the magic myself, I began to use it throughout my education. I relied on that trick so much, I used it all the way through passing legal exams in two countries, systems, and languages; changing careers; and writing this book itself.

I'd stand at the doorway of the exam hall and close my eyes. I'd feel in my bones, cells, and skin how it was to sit in the exam hall. I imagined gripping the pen in my hand and moving it avidly across the paper. But most importantly, I felt how good it was to close the final page of the exam paper and know I had passed. I charged my heart, pen, and every cell within me that this would be the outcome.

I didn't realize the impact of our sensations on manifestation — the magic trick from the athlete on *Blue Peter*! I'm grateful to that section of the program that day, because it equipped me with a tool I've since used throughout my life. It's here that I'd like to share with you both the science and the sensuality to support that system.

The Manifesting Recipe: The Law of Attraction Using the Senses

Manifesting is the meeting point of science, spirit, and sensuality. It's an age-old concept, spanning different cultures and countries, through rituals and prayers. Since popular manifestation books like *The Science of Getting Rich* (by Wallace Wattles, 1910), *The Master Key System* (Charles F. Haanel, 1916), and *The Secret* (Rhonda Byrne, 2006), manifesting through the Law of Attraction has become more accessible and gained much traction worldwide.

Simply put, the Law of Attraction teaches us that our thoughts determine our reality and we attract what we think. Science and medicine have since been able to provide research to support the impact of our thoughts; if you're interested in exploring this further, neuroscientist Dr. Tara Swart includes important information in her book, *The Source: Open Your Mind, Change*

Your Life.[1] The book explores the scientific principles underpinning the Law of Attraction.

Dr Swart shares two functions that are working in the brain when we manifest. The first is *selective attention*, during which the thalamus is activated; this is the part of the limbic system that manages the brain's filtering of all the information we receive from our senses and the world around us. It allows us to pay attention to what's important and to filter out what isn't. For example, if you're reading a book on a busy train, you might filter out some of the sounds of the tracks and people you hear, the advertisements or flurry of things past the window you see, and maybe even the smells around you – to focus on the words you're reading while keeping an ear out for the announcement of your stop.

The thalamus is the center of our senses that gathers information and redirects it. Call it the 'bouncer' or 'doorway' for our sacred sense messengers; information lines up at the door of the thalamus, which decides what gets in and what doesn't. This is particularly important in a world where we're bombarded with information and sensory stimuli.

How does the bouncer choose what makes the selection? It lets in what it recognizes, what is safe, and what is useful. When we learn this, we can begin to appreciate the deeply unconscious processes that are happening from moment to moment within us.

Through the power of manifestation and selectively
focusing our thoughts, we can begin to train
our brains to recognize and draw in the sensory
information that previously slipped our attention.

Once the lucky few pieces of information we've received through the senses are through the door, the second function Dr. Swart mentions in her book is value tagging, which takes the sensory information and decides how important it is.

If you've spent until now focused on your career, but deep down you also want a life partner, it's likely your thalamus will have filtered out potential partners to focus on potential promotions because it's tagged more value to that form of information. But when you learn that manifestation is a sensual practice and begin to use the technique to visualize and sense with your whole body what your future partner will feel like, it may be that in a few months, something happens: Someone at work you never noticed before is wearing a delicious scent. It draws your curiosity, and you hold your attention a little longer than usual with that person through the week. This time, your thalamus unconsciously recognizes them from your visualization process and lets in the sensory information. The potential partner picks up on this longer-than-usual attention and walks toward you to strike up a conversation in the staff social later that week.

In refocusing on what we truly want, we can consciously 'tag' new sensory information and give it a value-added VIP wristband to get through the bouncer at the door.

This is why it's called the Law of Attraction: As you open the doors of perception, you embark on a deeply sensual process and cultivate the power to be in the driver's seat of your life.

Exploring the Unmanifest

To get what you want, you must know what you need.

It sounds so simple, but to bring the unmanifest into the manifest requires having clarity around what we want. This can be difficult, especially if we don't see ourselves as worthy of our desire or we just don't know where to begin. In the next chapters, we'll examine some of the Tantric and scientific theory around manifestation, including energetic resonance, the manifesting center of the body, and seven practical steps to manifest through the Sensual Rivermap.

First, one of the key aspects of manifestation lies in the power of the mind's eye to bring into focus what we're manifesting through visualization. In Chapter 4, we came across *Ajna chakra*. This center is housed in the head, eyes, and a pea-size pineal gland that produces melatonin, a derivative of serotonin, which is created when we sleep. This plays a role in our dreams, visions, near-death experiences, and psychedelic experiences through the synthesis of dimethyltryptamine (DMT), a structure that resembles natural neurotransmitters and produces internal visions. The sixth *chakra* is sometimes mistaken to be the forehead because of its popularized name of the 'third eye'; however, its location is actually the conjunction point between the left and right hemispheres of the brain, so it's more in the center of the head.[2]

Ajna means 'to perceive and to command.' We use our two eyes to see the world around us, but we use our 'third' eye to sense the world around us. Many paths and traditions have referred to this center as the one of mysticism and the soul, which is why it is often anointed. In Tantra, this is known as the *cave of Brahma* or the *command center*.

In mythology, Shiva is often depicted sending out a lightning bolt from the *Ajna chakra* to depict the great power of resting in our mind and thoughts, as well as the projection of those thoughts with concentrated focus out into the world. You may see the third eye visually depicted on Tantric deities to symbolize this key to all processes of consciousness, including our intuition, insight, memory, perception, impression, and dreams.

In the first line of Adi Shankaracharya's renowned hymn, 'Soundarya Lahari' (translating to 'waves of beauty'), from around 800 CE, it says, 'If Shiva is united with Shakti, he is able to create. If he is not, he is incapable even of stirring.'[3]

Ajna chakra is the meeting point of *ida* and *pingala nadis* (the major rivers carrying energy through the body), representing *shakti* (left) and *shiva* (right). For this reason, it's the spiritual center where you can experience union of the body, mind, and spirit, as well as the drawing together of the unmanifest (pure potential) and the manifest (material world), and of *shiva* and *shakti* energies. This is where duality dissolves and creative potential is birthed.

As you manifest and bring your focus and vision habitually to this center, it will reshape the neural structure of your brain. This is what's known in neuropsychological Hebbian theory as neuroplasticity, where the 'neurons which fire together wire together.'[4]

Let's explore what happens here.

Manifestation as a Sensuous Process

Visualization is powerful, but on its own, it isn't enough. To connect our sensuality to manifestation, we need to see not only what we're manifesting, but also feel it through our senses. We need to think about how it looks, sounds, tastes, feels, and smells. We need to consider its vibration.

Everything has a vibration – even items that seem solid, like the seat you're sitting on or the home you live in. If you zoom in, you'll see it's made up of atoms vibrating in a certain frequency.

There are millions of frequencies in the universe: There's the one that makes the chair you sit on, and there's also your own unique vibration that makes you *you*.

> *The process of connecting to our sensations gives us a pathway to connect to our energetic vibration. Each interaction, home, career, ambition, and emotion has a particular energetic vibration or frequency. In the process of manifestation, we're reverse-engineering by tapping into the sensation we'll be experiencing when we have, achieve, experience, or acquire what we're manifesting.*

As we close our eyes and visualize, we need to tune in to the feeling associated with it, be it satisfaction, joy, health, or love, and how it feels in our body. It might feel like warmth, relaxation in the muscles, or brightness in the heart. By bringing ourselves into this frequency through engineering our visualization with sensations, we begin to attract the people, opportunities, and potential that *are* that frequency. This is known as *energetic resonance*.

When you resonate with something, you're in sync with it. When you don't resonate with something, it feels contradictory, out of balance, or in disagreement with you. For example, in music, if all the notes vibrate on a similar frequency, they will harmonize and be in resonance with each other. If someone has a suggestion for a plan over the weekend and you disagree with it, you might feel a knot in your stomach and not resonate with it. Or, if you walk into a room where there are lots of stressed people, you may feel that stress, even without talking to them. Your personal vibration influences what's happening around you, and the people you're around the most are also influencing your vibration.

How we think, feel, and act around certain situations or people will tell us how 'in tune' or resonant we are. The more we bring in the power of visualization, the more powerful we become as manifesters.

The Seven Steps of Manifesting

You can use your *kundalini shakti* to power up the manifestation process in your body. The Sensual Rivermap is a powerful channel for the process of manifestation. Since the microcosm (the inner landscape of the body) represents the macrocosm (the wider universe), I have broken the seven steps of manifesting into each of the *chakras.*

> Shiva *lives at the crown as unmanifest potential, ideas, and dreams. Shakti lives at the root and pelvis, where our manifestations are birthed out into the world. The idea is to channel your* kundalini shakti — *the sexual creative energy, along with your intention, through every cell of the body!*

It can be top down, as we'll explore here, or bottom up, as we'll explore through the Sensual Sex Magic[5] practice at the end of this chapter (see p.201). It may help you to think about your life in different areas when you work to manifest; this will allow you to become more specific about your visualizations and sensations.

You can use the following categories and repeat steps 1–7. For now, choose one particular theme to work with as you go through the steps.

▼ **Personal journey:** how you feel about yourself (physical, mental, emotional, spiritual, sensual, health)

▼ **Work:** any job, business, working environment, career goal

▼ **Connections:** your friendships and family

▼ **Love and sex:** your romantic relationships

▼ **Hobbies:** any interests or projects you have going on

▼ **Home:** where you live and how you'd like that to look and feel

Step 1: Draw a Blank Canvas

Chakra: *Sahasrara*

Location: crown

Element: consciousness

The first step is drawing a blank canvas in the mind upon which to paint your senses. This allows you to empty your inner noise and start afresh. You can do this by bringing the body into an idle state and slowing down enough to focus on a single point. This might mean five minutes focusing on the breath; watching ocean waves, birds, or clouds move in the sky; seeing cars drive past as you wait for the bus; or lying down with eyes closed as you relax each part of the body in *savasana*. As you focus, you tune out the noise and tune in to the unmanifest potential of your blank manifesting canvas.

Step 2: Visualize

Chakra: *Ajna*

Location: third eye

Element: light

Next, bring to your mind's eye what you're manifesting with great specificity. It's the same way you type into a navigation app the name of a restaurant you want to go to, not just 'restaurant,' with a thousand options coming up. Compute in your visualization the specific sensory qualities of the things you're manifesting. If it's a house, it can't be any house. It needs to be the house you want. You need to imagine it with all your senses: its color, the number of rooms, the climate/environment, the sounds, whether it's in the city or country, etc.

If it feels difficult to imagine the exact details of what you're manifesting, you may find it helpful to create a vision board. You can either physically cut out pictures from newspapers or magazines, or use a picture stitcher on a phone or computer to pull together everything you'd like to include. Pinterest can be helpful in creating specific boards. You can then visualize and meditate on what you see in front of you to draw forward the sensations.

Step 3: Embody

Chakra: *Vishuddha*

Location: throat

Element: space/ether

This is one of the most important steps. Now that you've seen specifically what you're manifesting and explored it through the senses, it's time to explore how those sensations feel and how they get expressed. How would you move, sit, stand, and feel in your body? Can you really feel, in every inch of your body, just how relaxed you are sitting on the couch in your new living room? If what you want to manifest is a different career, how excited do you feel in the morning to wake up and head to the office? If it's a relationship, how comforting does it feel at the end of the day to come home and lie in the arms of your beloved as you fall asleep? When you sense, it's not about what you want – it's about connecting to who you are, as if you have it. Because you do!

Step 4: Believe

Chakra: *Anahata*

Location: heart

Element: air

It's all well to find, think about, and feel what we want, but if at our deepest core, we don't believe it's possible or that we're worthy of receiving it, our manifesting potential is blocked. This step is about self-love. To believe you're worthy of it, you can sit with the idea that you already are it or have it. This means the person who has these things exists within you, ready to be brought forward.

A helpful way to frame this in your thoughts is switching 'I want to have' or 'I would like to be' into 'I have' and 'I am.' For example, 'I have a beautiful house in (insert specific place, name, number, or street),' or, 'I am the founder of a successful business in XYZ,' or, 'I am healthy and love who I am.' The more you say it, the more you affirm it; the more you affirm it, the more you believe it, and your body starts to produce the magnetic energetic resonance required to attract what you want.

Step 5: Clear

Chakra: *Manipura*

Location: solar plexus

Element: fire

Sometimes we can hear our fears and our past more loudly than our newly formed beliefs. At this point, you may be called to burn and clear some of your past thoughts or beliefs. There are four helpful exercises that can help with clearing stagnancy in the mind, body, energy, and spirit:

▼ **Shaking the body:** Put on some music and shake the entire body from head to toe for three to five minutes minimum.

▼ **Cord-cutting meditation:** This is a visualization for cutting the energetic ties you have to a thing, place, person, or situation. You can find a meditation for this on the SOSA website (*see p.xxi*).

▼ **Ho'oponopono:** This is a Hawaiian forgiveness and reconciliation practice that uses a *mantra* to release negative emotions, thoughts, and experiences. The general form is 'I'm sorry, please forgive me, thank you, I love you.'

▼ **Connect to Kali:** The Tantric goddess of endings and beginnings can be accessed through meditation, *mantra*, or visualization (see Chapter 7).

Step 6: Charge

Chakra: *Svadhistana*

Location: between navel and genitals

Element: water

When life situations throw our energy off course, they pull us down to lower vibrational frequencies. This is where we cultivate our sensual *shakti* energy with the practices we have learned in this book. Here are some more things you can do to support this process:

▼ **Exercise:** Moving your body releases endorphins and reharmonizes your energy.

▼ **Change your environment:** You can go for a walk, work in a different room or spot, take a different route, shift perspective, and create new opportunities for resonance.

▼ **Work with gratitude:** Write down or speak out loud the people or things you are grateful for today.

▼ **Connect with nature:** Ground your feet into the earth, go for a swim, and come back to balance through the elements.

▼ **Practice yoga:** Yoga (Tantra Yoga in particular) works holistically across the spectrum of mind, body, energy, and spirit.

Step 7: Act

Chakra: *Mulhadhara*

Location: perineum (between anus and genitals)

Element: earth

It's easy to do this exercise once and hope for results, but manifestation is where vision meets aligned action. There is no manifestation goal too big or small, and you don't need the whole plan right away. Start by taking the first step to bring your visualizations into the manifest world through conscious action. Earth is made up of all the elements from the previous *chakras*, and represents bringing your idea or vision into reality. You can take the following steps.

Write down clear action points that will bring you from where you are now toward where you want to be. Then, write down dates for when you want your vision to manifest, and the actions you need to take. For example, 'In two months, I'm interviewing at my dream company. In one month, I've filled out five job applications. By the end of the year, I'm working my dream job.'

▼ Activity ▼

Sensual Sex Magic

Sensual sex magic is an incredible self-pleasure or dual cultivation practice that uses *shakti* energy for manifestation. Here's a ritual we share at SOSA.

1. Create a beautiful sacred space and relax your body by connecting to your senses.

2. Set an intention and begin to visualize it: Notice what it looks, smells, feels, sounds, and tastes like; notice the sensations in your body.

3. Slowly massage the body using oil, exploring the sensations that arise.

4. Begin to self-pleasure and pass your breath through each *chakra*. Breathe deeply in and out of each *chakra*, spending 1–3 minutes in each area and imagine the energy cultivating and swirling there. This time, move from the root all the way up to the crown (use the edging practice to pause if it becomes too much, to slow down the process).

5. In the root, imagine the foundation/smell of what you are manifesting.

6. In the sacral center, imagine the taste/flavor/style.

7. In the solar plexus, imagine what it looks like.

8. In the heart, imagine the feeling/sensation.

9. In the throat, imagine how it sounds.

10. In the third eye, bring all the senses together, fully embodied.

11. In the crown, release your intention into the universe (this may be through orgasm, but doesn't have to be).

12. Lie in *savasana* or just be still, so you can integrate and receive sensations of manifestation back from the universe. Call in love, protection, and guidance.

13. Journal the downloads you received.

Integration

1. For one minute after you wake up and one minute before you go to sleep, take time to connect to your manifesting vision.

2. Keep pictures of your vision board or affirmations in clear sight: on your desktop, phone background, tagged on the fridge or bathroom mirror, or placed anywhere you frequently go.

3. Set a ritual manifesting the month ahead in your diary — to release what's not needed and invite in what is (for example, at every new moon, on the first day of menstruation, or at the end of each month).

4. Try one of the practices and journal what you find.

Key Takeaways

~ Meeting the manifester within enables you to shape your life in the ways your soul desires.

~ Manifestation is the ability to move an energy into action and bring the unmanifest into the manifest. The process is greatly simplified when you connect to sensuality.

~ The Law of Attraction teaches that our thoughts determine our reality, and we attract what we think. Selective attention and value tagging are important aspects of working with the Law of Attraction.

~ The *Ajna chakra*, or third eye, can help us focus on what we are manifesting through the power of visualization.

~ Manifestation is a sensuous practice that can be approached with seven steps that take us through each *chakra*, from crown to root, to bring the unmanifest into manifest form.

~ To continue to live rooted in alignment with your vision, it's important to keep revisiting the seven steps. You can make use of the different categories and focus where you want your energy to flow the most.

CHAPTER 10

Meeting the Creative Within

Creativity is the language of your sensual soul. When you channel your sensual energy into creative living, you give it an avenue to speak and interact with the world.

Channeling sensuality into creativity doesn't mean you need to be a starving artist or professional poet. Creative living is available to each and every human. The way you dress, the walk you take to work, the arrangement of your home, the curiosity you demonstrate, and even how you cook and place food on a plate are all decisions that connect us with the creative spirit, *shakti*.

So many of us lose touch with our creative spirit in our formative years because we're told we can't draw, dance, sing, paint, etc. — as if creativity is only a skill for the gifted or a way to make money, and not a means of human expression as old as humankind. This cuts off an entire avenue of sensual expression in our adult years.

Creativity expresses all that is underneath the surface that hasn't quite made its way up into verbal form. It offers us a pathway to know ourselves on the most intimate levels. Most mystic paths, like Tantra, Sufism, or Kabbalah, share creativity as a means of connecting to the divine. As we'll explore in this chapter, anything you do to create draws you closer to knowing yourself as the creative spirit.

Shakti Circle Creativity

One evening I had wandered into the compound, looking for the circle. I stared up at the tall buildings kissed by the bright-black Beijing sky. That's when she found me. She was a Chinese lady making motions from afar: 'Hello, are you looking for the circle? You look lost. Follow me.'

I smiled, as kindness led me under the moonlight to where I needed to go. We gathered there, 20 people from all around the world, on the night of the eclipse. We sat silently in the circle of a dimly lit room, touched only by the soft glimmer of candlelight.

'Creativity,' the circle leader whispered. 'This is the topic today... you will introduce yourself and what it means to you.'

As if it were an AA meeting for the creatively averse, she started talking while a mental energy filled the silent room. 'We do not judge, we do not question, and we do not discuss,' she said, passing a white flower to the woman on her left, close to where I sat.

A magical microphone gave the power of voice to the holder, while the others listened without judgment. *If only these rules always governed conversation and creativity*, I thought.

Meanwhile, a lump formed in my throat. My father is a professionally trained Master of Fine Arts in sculpture, and I often found myself lost in the subject of creativity, with an enormous pressure to execute it with perfection. But how to express this feeling of creativity? It was like magic in a jar I kept locked inside my heart.

I looked up. I could see everyone on the other side of the circle, quickly searching inward, grateful for the extra time.

My turn soon came. 'Hi, my name is Henika and I think creativity comes as some kind of external being, one that comes and goes as a moment of inspiration, giving you only a moment to capture it before it moves through you to the next person.'

I passed the flower to the next woman. Relief. I listened carefully to the others, who described the creativity like a drug with which we all had varying degrees of experience. And we did. Some expressed never having a single dose, others tapped in and out of its hands, and a few concluded that every living moment is a creation and therefore creative.

But what was this circle? Why had we come there on the eve of the eclipse? What were we searching for? Connection, expression, union – and at its heart, I knew that was exactly what creativity offered.

Sensual Energy Is Creative Energy

If sensual and creative energy are two sides of the same coin, that coin is found in the second *chakra*, known as *Svadhistana*, which we encountered in Chapter 4. *Svadhistana* translates to the 'dwelling place of the self.' It's located three to four fingers below the belly button and rules the hips, sacrum, lower back, inner thighs, and lower abdomen. It regulates the flow of *prana* in the sexual organs, bladder, and kidneys. You can think of it as your inner watermill – churning water, excretory liquids, emotions, toxins, and sensual energy in and out of the body.

Let's take a closer look at the physical functions of these organs. If *Svadhistana* is the watermill, the bladder is a reservoir. The ureters carry urine away from the kidneys to the bladder, which acts to hold and control it there. Just like any body of water, it holds and absorbs what's put into it. A drop of ink bleeds into the cup of water it's dropped into. In the same way, the water in your body absorbs whatever you put into it – the glass of wine you had at dinner or the stress and frustration you may have felt just before that. The bladder stores what it needs to hydrate us, and excretes the physical and emotional toxins in urine through the urethra, the tube carrying urine from the bladder out of our body and into the toilet.

The link between the water functions of the body, our pelvic floor, and our emotions has long been known in Ayurveda and Traditional Chinese Medicine, and is now confirmed in scientific studies[1] which share that psychological and emotional factors have a profound influence on the pelvic floor and liver, as well as bladder dysfunction. All of these organs soak up unprocessed emotions, trauma, and experiences over the course of our lives.

The same way a watermill takes in water and turns its fans to generate energy, *Svadhistana* turns a wheel with our inner waters to generate creative *shakti* energy for our *pranamaya kosha*, the energetic layer of the body that feeds all our cells and organs with vital life force. This means that charging the sensual energy in the body also charges our creative energy, and vice versa.

So, put a piece of music on and dance like no one's watching, dust off the paints in your cupboard, and sing to your heart's content each morning in the shower – it'll not only bring you more deeply into your body and your emotions, but it'll draw you deeper into the flow of your sensuality.

The Psychology of Creativity

When I returned to the UK after several years in the East, I became curious about creativity as a form of therapeutic expression and began to study art therapy at my local university. While I studied, I volunteered and worked in addiction rehabilitation clinics, for schools, governments, and even at army events for personnel who served abroad.

It became clear to me that emotion, creativity, and sensual living are intrinsically linked, particularly when we don't have the language to express what might be stored in our unconscious memory – in the form of early experiences or traumatic events and emotions we haven't yet processed. What doesn't get expressed gets repressed and plays out in different coping mechanisms or repetitions.

The founder of psychoanalysis, Sigmund Freud, described an unconscious mental process by which instinctual, socially unacceptable sexual energy and libido are transferred to a non-instinctual, socially acceptable activity via a process called sublimation. (Similar to the sublimation we've been exploring in the SENSFUL Method!) Freud believed that sublimation of unsatisfied libido was behind the creation of great art and literature.[2] This way, inner repression can be reworked subconsciously and reemerge through creativity. It's an adaptive way of regulating repressed or overwhelming emotions.

In addition, psychologist Abraham Maslow described creativity as an act of self-actualization and a 'kind of permission to be ourselves'. He describes the hallmark of creative outcome as 'great bursts of emotion and enthusiasm.' He later theorized that creativity is inhibited when we lose touch with our emotions and drives. He described creativity as a way of being wholly true to who you are and what you feel.[3]

Famous creators have mentioned emotions as an integral part of the creative process, as motivators, inhibitors, and a kind of building material from which the creations are made.[4] As emotions are energy in motion, all our sensations carry with them potential for creative expression. For example, if we express fear through our art or creative expression, then Tantra would say what we create transmutes or sublimates the charge of our fear. It is discharged from one place and form to another, moving from inside the body to outside, where its charge is released and transformed.

Social psychologist James Averill has shared how creativity gives individuals this agency in processing, understanding, and regulating emotions, as well as becoming creators of their own emotional experience and way of expressing it.[5] In psychology, agency refers to a sense of control and the capacity to influence our behavior and have faith in our ability to handle situations. Through creativity, we can become the empowered 'agents' of processing our inner landscape and deepening our sensuality.

Sensual Art Forms Over the Ages

Since ancient times, we humans have been touched by the double-sided coin of sensuality and creativity — whether we're feeling, expressing, or witnessing them. Creative, sensuous forces have traveled their way through the shaking hips of belly dance in the Middle East, the sacred dance forms represented on temples in India, the Xibelani dance and its shaking skirts in South Africa, and the fine arts of courtesans and geishas in the Far East, as well as many other cultures around the world.

In ancient civilizations, sensuality was not suppressed or seen as dirty, reserved for red-light districts and secrets. Rather, it formed a bridge between daily life and the divine, forging a path to connect to and express rather than repress our life-force energy. It was used to inspire great creativity, poetry, art, music, and dance.

In India, communities would gather in temples and royal courts to receive the wisdom of sensuality as it expressed itself through the highly skilled sacred temple dancers, and later, through the country's courtesans. Those who gathered to receive the channeling often went with a question and, in return, were bestowed with great wisdom and messages from the divine. The same way someone might go to a priest or spiritual sage for advice, people would go to the sacred dancers to receive from their movements the secret whisperings of the divine that moved through the sensual artists' bodies, poetry, music, dance, and voices.

Sacred temple dance gave access to the cosmic answers of the universe. In a society where answers are predominantly formed, asked, and answered by the mind, books, and Google, this form of communication with a higher power and creative forces through nonverbal transmission can be hard to grasp — so, let's take a look back to the origins.

The Agamas are a set of sacred doctrines and treatises that share traditions of divine worship with great detail, from devotional practices, meditations, mantras, and temple buildings to visual representations of the divine, sacred geometry, and esoteric and exoteric worship. In the Agamas, music and dance are set out as key routes to connect to the divine. The Agamas are split into three doctrines for three distinctive spiritual paths, which still exist in India and across Sanatana Dharma (the precolonial name for Hinduism) today.

1. The Vaishnava Agamas are for followers of the god Vishnu, sometimes known by his avatar, Krishna. These practices share the path of *bhakti* (devotion), and go by the name Vaishnavism.

2. The Shaiva Agamas are for followers of Shiva, whom we previously learned about. This path goes by the name Shaivism.

3. The Shakta Agamas are for followers of Shakti, and her many manifestations; the sect goes by the name *Shaktism*.

The Legacy of Sensual Dance in India

Owing to this foundation, India was once a land rich with dancers in service to the divine. In Madhur Gupta's book, *Courting Hindustan: The Consuming Passions of Iconic Women Performers in India*,[6] we learn that in South India, temple dancers were known as *devadasis*, meaning 'servants of the divine,' or *maharis*, meaning 'the greatest women.' They were often married to the temple deities whom they looked after and channeled their crafts from.

This ritual and sacred dance form with the divine later transformed into *nautch*, a court art coming from the term *nach*, meaning 'to dance.' In *Nautch Girls of the Raj*, Pran Nevile shares how these dancers were esteemed with a high degree of social sophistication and elevated status in society. He writes, 'The nautch girl was no ordinary woman of pleasure, she had refined manners, a ready wit and poetry in her blood, she embodied a splendid synthesis of different cultures and dance forms, the classical and the popular.'[7]

In North India, highly skilled courtesans were known as *tawaifs* and were predominant in the Mughal dynasty between the 16th and 19th centuries. They were a core part of society and had a high status. Their intimate ties with notable figures such as the maharajas were often polygamous in nature. This was a social norm similar to the relationships between courtesans and emperors of the Far East.

Nevile goes on to describe how Indian poets sang praises to temple dancers; the Puranas highlight them as a symbol of good luck. Also, Buddhist literature testifies to the high esteem they held in society and shares the different forms they appear in through the ages, from *apsaras* (celestial beings), to *devadasis* (spiritual dancers), to *tawaifs* (cultured courtesans), to *nautch* girls (dancers in professional troupes).

The divine manifests in the heavenly dances and sensual archetypes across civilization, in the history and cultures from India to Greece and everywhere in between. Sensual artistry was a form of creative artistry that connects us to *shakti* and spirit. This leaves us with the question: Where did that sensual artistry go, and what can we do to reclaim it?

What Happened to the Sensual Arts?

Let's take a closer look back to the dancing *devadasis* of India and what happened to them.

The British East India Company first established its trade point in Surat, a city in my home region of Gujarat in Western India, in 1608. The Mughal emperor gave a royal permit to the company to establish factories on this coast; by 1615, they had freedom to trade across the Mughal territory.

After the decisive victory in the Battle of Plassey, the East India Company began to rule across India in 1757. During this time, the *nautch* girl was ingrained in society and had a special position, even among the English *sahibs*. A century later, the Government of India Act 1858 called to liquidate the British East India Company and transfer its functions to the British Crown to begin its official rule over India. This included the land that is now Pakistan and Bangladesh, and excluded a few places where other European nations had holdings – such as Goa, which was ruled by Portugal, and Pondicherry, which was ruled by France.

This commenced the era of the Raj, or British rule over India. As the Raj reached the shores of India, it brought petite-bourgeois values, and missionaries to set up new forms of education and indoctrination. *Devadasis* and the ancient sensual arts were considered 'repulsive and immoral' by these standards. Temple dancers and courtesans were misunderstood by the new rulers, who were not familiar with the culture. From the misogynistic and culturally prudish viewpoint of the Raj, *devadasis* were criminals; many of them were forced to shift from their reputable status as divine dancers into prostitution.

After 2,500 years, what had once been a sacred and skilled creative art was sullied by oppressive misunderstandings and converted into slavery, crime, and poverty. As the land was pillaged for its riches and jewels, so were its sacred traditional art forms, temples, and dancers. The long history of sensuality was weeded out of the lands, along with the crown jewels. Courtesan culture and sacred temple dance in India had come to an end.

Even if dancers, musicians, and other sacred artists and artisans were highly skilled, they were deemed to be of immoral character. The educated and highly esteemed high-status Indians who'd once embraced *devadasi* culture, inviting them to dance at their weddings and keeping a place for them in their family paintings, were also influenced to please the colonizing forces and petitioned to end the tradition.

The sacred sensual arts transformed into the barbarous arts; finally, what was once the country's prized cultural jewel came to an end through a series of laws that declared courtesan and *devadasi* culture illegal. For generations, the expression of sensuality in India became shameful and dangerous, and still remains so in the 21st century.

So, what's left of the ancient sacred sensual arts? Traces of ancient temple dance are still seen in classical dance forms such as Bharatanatyam and Odissi, though not in the same way. While temple dancers are no longer the norm, you can still see temples in India with walls covered in the sculptures of *apsaras* and dancers with their waists and breasts bared, documenting the devotional days of sensuality as a way of communing with the divine; this is notable throughout the beautiful temples in Khajuraho, India.

I spoke with art historian Manju Gautum about the historical perspectives of nude figures that still adorn temples and paintings from the precolonial era. She told me these are not erotic, perverse, or sexual figures, but rather, representative of the times in which they were made – a time when *saris* were worn wrapped around the waist, breasts were free of bras, and sensuality was a divine transmission carried through the sacred sensual creative arts.

Let's meet the goddesses of creativity now, and learn some practices to reclaim sensual artistry!

Saraswati: Goddesses of Creativity

The sacredness of creativity is celebrated through Saraswati, the goddess of knowledge, music, art, speech, eloquence, melody, wisdom, and learning, who is depicted sitting poised on a swan, with her four arms holding a book, a rosary, a pot of water, and a stringed instrument called a *veena*.

The name *Saraswati* derives from the word *saras*, meaning 'pooling water,' and *surasa-vati*, meaning 'the one with plenty of water.' Her name evolves its meaning in the Vedas, as 'a flow of water, speech, and knowledge that purifies,' and lends itself to the essence of her flow, which is embodied through creativity.

In mythology, Saraswati was the creator god Brahma's partner, and his *shakti*. She invites us learn, create, and evolve. She is also the deity of the river Saraswati, one of the seven holy rivers first mentioned in the Rig Veda. This river represented a pathway to the heavens – and Saraswati, in her creative, alluring ways, represented the route through creativity. She draws us back to the powerful flow of our inner and outer waters and their creative potential.

Tantric Saraswati: Matangi

In Chapter 5 you met Matangi, one of the Dasa Mahavidyas. She is a creative, rebellious goddess who invites us to embrace our inner 'weirdness,' uniqueness, and darkness as a birthing ground for creativity.

She holds mastery over the arts, like Saraswati, but Matangi is the outcast goddess. She is often associated with pollution and that which is inauspicious, including the things that make us cringe and feel disgusted. She invites us to explore these parts of ourselves as a vehicle for expansion and creativity.

She is represented with emerald skin, wearing a bright red *sari*. She holds the *veena* and is pictured with a parrot, a noose, a goad, and a club. She invites us to embrace all the unique aspects of ourselves we might reject, and weave them into the tapestry of who we are. In creativity, she encourages us to push the boundaries of what is 'normal' and acceptable, to find the expression that will connect to the deep truths of who we are.

▼ Activities ▼

Tantra Sacred Dance

The following practice is from my teacher, Ma Deva Vibha. Tantra Sacred Dance is a way to fall in love with yourself through movement. In each dance, you are invited not to perform for others, but to feel the many sensations and energies dancing within. Through the dance, you are invited to channel, intuit, and connect to your higher power – and receive, in the way temple dancers once did, communication with universal consciousness and *parashakti* through the vessel of your body.

1. Setting: Create your temple as a devotional space in your home or in nature, where you feel free. You can choose to do this alone with your own inner witnessing presence, but originally, Tantra Sacred Dance was meant to be done with witnesses who receive wisdom from your dance. Being seen in our highest potential can be a transformational and healing experience.

2. Music: Put on sacred music that resonates with your heart. Visit the SOSA website (*see p.xxi*) for sacred dance music recommendations.

3. Body positioning: Step your feet hip width or slightly wider apart; bend through your knees gently and connect your feet to the earth. Place one hand on your heart and one hand on *Svadhistana chakra* (four fingers below belly button). Close your eyes and take a moment to arrive in your body.

4. Intention: Bring to your heart a question you have in your life, or something you'd like to heal – or explore a vision for something you'd like to manifest. You can also choose to embody a goddess or archetype. Whatever you choose, keep it in your vision but don't let it keep you in your head; allow it to dissolve and flow through your body.

5. *Shakti*: Begin rocking the hips and pelvis back and forth to evoke *kundalini shakti*.

6. Flow: Move slowly, like a leaf blowing in the wind. Tantra Sacred Dance is a slow-moving meditation in which, rather than learning steps or performing, you're moved by the sensual energy of *kundalini shakti* within. It's less about moving and doing, and more about being moved and receiving.

7. Time: If you're with others, dance the length of a song or set a time of five to 10 minutes per person. If alone, you can do this for as long as you would like to explore.

8. Witness: If with others, the people in the temple are witnessing you in your highest potential and noticing the lessons or messages they receive from your dance. Sit in a circle and go around one by one to share these messages. It's not about watching, complimenting, or criticizing the dance – it's about the transmission from the sacred dance to the witness. If alone, take a few minutes to lie down or meditate on what you have received; then, pick up a journal and write down your downloads.

Free-Flow Writing

Writing is an incredible way of exploring the unconscious mind and expressing it. If we apply the phrase 'dance as if no one is watching' to writing, we'll find that we can experience a free flow of our conscious and unconscious thought pouring onto the pages.

You don't need to worry about grammar, sentence structure, spelling, others' judgments, or anything else. You only need to put pen to paper and experience the incredible shifts in energy and transmutation of emotions and sensual energy from your body onto the paper.

1. Environment: Sit down in a space where you won't be disturbed.

2. Time: Set a time for free-flowing; start with five minutes before moving to 10–15+.

3. Space: Open a blank page in your journal. This exercise is most effective with pen to paper.

4. Prompt: This could be a single subject that's on your mind. You can also find a list of journal prompts on the SOSA website, choose an image to respond to, or simply see what emerges on the empty page.

5. Integrate: Make sure to put your pen down when the time ends, and go back right away or later in the day to read what has emerged. See it as a way of making connections, engaging in uninhibited expression, and exploring your inner world. (Remember, don't go back and edit!)

Therapeutic Art Making

Therapeutic art making is not about creating the perfect picture; it lifts the burden of needing to be a talented artist or producing a final product that has value or requires skill. The focus is on the journey of making itself.

Therapeutic art can be done by yourself, to better understand your inner landscape, and it often draws out unconscious expression. It can also be done with a professionally trained art therapist to make sense of your unconscious expression in a therapeutic setting.

There are many therapeutic art exercises available. One is drawing and interpreting mandalas, which are used as a meditative tool to explore the micro- and macrocosm in Tantra and Buddhism.

We share a guided Mandala Drawing and Interpreting workshop with more of a historical context on the SOSA website.

Mandala Drawing and Interpretation

1. Space: Find a quiet space to call your own.

2. Template: Using a compass, draw a circle with several circles inside; divide the circle into six or eight sections, using a ruler to draw three or four lines. The more lines, the more intricate the mandala. You can download a template from the SOSA website.

3. Intention: Set an intention with what is on your mind, or a particular question you might be exploring. You may also simply flow and see what comes.

4. Draw: The key is starting in one section and drawing the same pattern in each section of the line all the way around that line. For example, if I draw an 'm' shape on the inner circle, the whole line of the inner circle will have 'm' repeated on it. You can change patterns, as long as each section in that line replicates the pattern. Don't worry if it's not exact – it's more about the process.

5. Meditate: The repetitive nature of replicating a single pattern draws us into deep states of meditation.

6. Interpretation: When you're finished, look at your mandala and practice word association. Quickly, write down as many shapes and colors as you see. After this, write down what you associate with those shapes and colors. For example, if you see orange, you might associate it with passion, heat, fire, warmth, fruit, etc.

7. Title: Choose two words you wrote down that resonate most with you. Add the title 'The Mandala of X and X,' including the two words. Journal on what this is reflecting to you.

Integration

1. What creative activities do you enjoy (this is different to 'What are you good at?')?

2. What has your relationship with creativity been like over the course of your life? (It often reflects our relationship with sensuality.)

3. Do you have any creative practices in your culture/area/ community you can get involved with more deeply (such as a vocal ensemble, dance class, craft group, etc.)?

4. Try one of the practices from the chapter and reflect on what you find.

Key Takeaways

~ Creativity is the language of your sensual soul, and it's available to all of us.

~ *Svadhistana chakra* is the dwelling place of the self, and is associated with creativity and sensuality.

~ Because emotions are energy in motion, all our sensations carry with them the potential for creative expression.

~ In ancient civilizations, sensuality was not suppressed or seen as dirty. Rather, it formed a bridge between daily life and the divine, and was used to inspire great creativity, poetry, art, music, and dance.

~ The Agamas are a set of sacred doctrines and treatises that share traditions of divine worship with great detail, including the creation of sacred art.

~ Temple dance was once a revered art form in India, but colonization reduced it from its high status to something shameful and barbarous.

~ The goddess Saraswati and her Tantric counterpart, Matangi, help us bravely to claim and harness our creative expression and authentic self.

CHAPTER 11

Meeting the Desire Within

In the ancient sacred text of the Mahabharata, it says, 'Desire is the essence of life.' To desire is to be alive. When desire ceases, life ceases.

There was a desire that brought you into human form, and desire courses through you as you inhabit that human form. There's the simple desire that lifts your feet from your bed to touch the earth each morning, and there's the desire to nourish your body and engage your mind and senses. Desire is the source of all action and inaction; it is the seed of your needs and choices. Consequently, it is the seed of who you are and how you choose to live your life.

Up until now, we've learned how to channel our sensual energy outward to manifest and create. In this chapter, we'll learn how we can channel the same energy inward, for our own fulfilment and expression.

Darkness and Desire

In some of the darker days I described earlier in this book, I had lost my *iccha shakti*: my will and desire. This first manifested in my relationship, where I began searching for the spark that fizzled out like a flailing firework and left me in darkness. Then, with that dark night's sky, I began to search for the lost spark inside myself.

I've learned that, yes, desire is raging hot passion, steamy showers, and electric connection – but it's also the will to take your feet out of bed in the morning, to make a cup of coffee and let the sun shine on your face, to contribute to society and live a meaningful life.

I remember not having the words to express my desire, and slowly that desire and its roots became weaker and weaker. Here then, we learn to give voice to desire as a channel for it to express and strengthen itself again.

The Seeds of Desire

Desire and expression are deeply intertwined. If desire is the seed, then expression makes up the roots, action is its flower, and completion its fruits.

This is the nature of who we are: hearts, minds, and bodies with a longing to satisfy that which we desire. The seeds are always there. It is only in the moments when we do not acknowledge these seeds that we cut off the natural life cycle of desire.

Desires that are repressed remain active within us, seeking expression or gratification, even if they are denied. The natural desire of any seed is to sprout – and no matter how much we try to hide from, push down, or fight it, it will do its best to find its way through the concrete of doubt toward expression.

Most humans feel desire, but many humans do not learn how to create healthy conversations with desire as a tool for spiritual and sensual evolution. This keeps our desires pressed down and creates conflict, disharmony, and dis-ease in the body. For this reason, desire can often emerge as cravings, addictions, greed, compulsion, controlling behavior, disorders, or aversions that tug at our minds and bodies. This very human experience is often villainized across many spiritual paths, as it causes distractions and fluctuations of the mind.

Many of us are left questioning our desires, not feeling worthy of them, or feeling guilty for having them at all. But desire is not something we *have*. It is something we innately and naturally *are*. If we are alive, then we desire to exist. When we deny desire, we deny the truth of our existence.

This is why expression and desire go hand in hand; they hold a conversation in our bodies and minds that helps us connect more deeply on our journey — as long as we don't treat them as foes to be driven out or pushed into repression. Expressing our desires helps us to create a healthy channel for sensual energy to flow — and where desire flows, sensuality goes. We may believe that we need to fulfill our desire, but sometimes, expression and acceptance of desire can create a strong-enough channel for sensual satisfaction.

Giving Voice to Desire: The Anatomy of Expression

We can experience deeply intimate sensual experiences by sharing, expressing, listening to, and understanding our own and each other's desires. Our voice creates a vibration that echoes around our body and penetrates the world. Our ears listen to the vibrations around us and receive the desires of others. This is also an intimately internal process that involves the expression and acknowledgment of desire within. Conversation, after, all is the two-way dance of both speaking and listening.

The expression of desire, when it is both spoken and heard, leads to wholeness, satisfaction, and completion in our lives. Its home is in our communication center, *Vishuddha chakra*.

Vishuddha translates to 'purification.' Purification is the process of extracting something from a substance. In this case, that substance is our soul's desire. From our desires, we extract our needs, our boundaries, and our choices. Purification is also referred to in the process of making something spiritually or ceremonially appropriate. *Vishuddha* is therefore also rooted in the concept of *satya*, meaning 'truth,' which is what purifies.

If we live our truth as we speak, our voice becomes the vehicle of our soul and sensuality. As Mahatma Gandhi said, 'Happiness is when what you think, what you say, and what you do are in harmony.'

Vishuddha is located in our neck, throat, shoulders, tongue, mouth, and ears, which are all essential components of expression. Its element is space. It affects our thyroid, which plays a crucial role in regulating our metabolism and producing hormones essential for our growth and development. It also influences the larynx, which has three important functions: producing sound for speech, protecting the airways, and controlling airflow during breathing. At the center of the larynx are the vocal cords. They're made of muscles covered by a thin layer of mucosa.[1] When we breathe in, the muscles pull cartilage to open our airways; when we speak, they close. Our throat is a physical, emotional, and energetic guard and gateway to the space of our inner world.

Vagina to Voice and Back

When viewed from above, there's a right and left fold of the vocal cords that form a V shape. This mirrors another gateway to our inner world: the yoni (Sanskrit for 'vulva, womb, reproductive organs, cervix, and vagina').

The anatomical structure of the voice box and the yoni are incredibly similar. Both have a hammock-like set of diaphragmatic muscles that move in tandem with respiration.

Notice as you breathe in, there's a subtle expansion in your throat, lungs, and pelvic floor; and as you exhale, there's a subtle contraction in all three places. These are your three diaphragms. In Latin, the word cervix refers to the neck, and in contemporary English, cervix is used to describe the 'neck' of the womb. You only need to hear the roaring sounds of childbirth, during which the cervix dilates, to begin to understand how the voice facilitates the cervix to open. This also explains why, during intense orgasm, involuntary and guttural sounds often accompany the experience.

In the clinical studies of ENT specialist Dr. Jean Abitbol and gynecologist Dr. Beatrice Abitbol, they found that the hormonal changes and fluctuations throughout a person's biological lifespan affect both their vocal-fold and vaginal tissues. Dr. Jean took smear tests of singers' vocal folds at different stages of the menstrual cycle and then sent them to his wife, Dr. Beatrice, who did cervical smears. When they put the two sets of slide images together, they couldn't tell the difference between the vocal folds and the vagina.[2]

For a visual representation of the striking similarities between the vocal cords and *yoni*, take a look at the work by artist Luisa Alexandre on the SOSA website.

Both speaking and orgasm are powered by rhythmic muscular pulses, so the cervix and the pelvic floor are inextricably linked to the vocal cords and larynx. If you have a penis, you'll be interested to know that, for all bodies, the pelvic floor and voice are connected by the vagus nerve, the wandering nerve that's stimulated and relaxed by all yogic and Tantric practices!

Previously, it was thought that this main nerve didn't reach the pelvic floor but we know now that it does. In fact, it 'wanders' up through the cervix, pelvic bowl and uterus. It then carries nerve impulses from those regions through the abdomen, digestive system, and an opening in the thoracic diaphragm, boogies through the chest cavity, splits into two pathways to shimmy through the larynx, up the neck and into the brain. And wanders back down. Vagina to voice and back.[3]

Over the course of our lives, each time our voice and desire are shut down, the message is stored and mirrored in both the pelvis and throat.[4] The immediate physical response to trauma, whether in an isolated incident or over the course of time, is known as *body armoring* and can be a physical, emotional, or energetic barrier we unconsciously put up in these areas to prevent further pain and protect ourselves. This is similar to *granthis* (psychic and energetic knots and tangles), which we explored in Chapter 6.

Excess tension in our respiratory diaphragm and pelvic floor can restrict oxygen intake and carbon-dioxide output, which creates a starvation response and cuts off sensation, communication, and control in the area. In our throats, this can feel like a lump or heaviness, or fluctuation of the voice as whiny, shrill, or changing in pitch. In the pelvis, this can feel like tension, numbness, or pain. This can lead to vaginismus, which occurs when the vaginal muscles tighten up automatically in reaction to penetration. In the penis, this can lead to erectile dysfunction.

Armoring helps protect us from further pain but also stops us from deeper connection to our desires, pleasure, and expression. When sensations are ignored and not responded to, they can turn into pain; when pain is not responded to, it turns into numbness and armoring. But like any muscle, we can release the knots and tensions, and bring *shakti* and sensation back to the dried-up rivers of energy, the *nadis*. We can rebuild communication through targeted exercise of the muscles and create space for conversation with and expression of our desires.

There are four keys to do this: breath, sound, movement, and safety. We can access these keys through conversation, therapy, embodiment, Tantra Yoga, *mantra*, *pranayama*, bodywork, and massage, which we will explore in this chapter's practices.

When a river refills its currents, it draws up through its force the sediments from its riverbeds. In this way, when our sensual *shakti* energy reaches and begins to replenish any area of our physical, emotional, or energetic body that was previously dry, we may feel the sediment of all that was pressed down, building up or blocking sensual flow. This can emerge in different sensations throughout the body and can also release different energies through motion, anger, tears, laughter, pain, and frustration, to name a few. We can work to heal and give love to the parts of ourselves that emerge, through steady regular practices that keep energy flowing. Where our focus goes, energy flows.

> *Using your voice to express what is within — whether it is pain, pleasure or desire — can help to evoke, release, and cultivate the sensual* shakti *within.*

Desire as a Pillar of Life

In Sanskrit, *kama* means 'desire.' *Kama* is recognized as the source of action, creation, and procreation. Initially, *kama* was regarded as the 'animating principle' of the cosmos in the Vedas, the largest body of ancient Sanskrit texts informing Hinduism.

The Rig Veda shares a hymn of creation:

> *In the beginning desire descended on it, that was the primal seed, born of the mind.*[5]

It refers to a primal life force, energy, or *prana* responsible for creation. From darkness and nothingness, *kama* was the seed from which the universe was created. Without running into too much of a chicken and egg argument, it suggests that desire was the first act of consciousness from which the material world was born. This suggests that everything, including ourselves, was born of desire.

Given its importance, a few centuries after the Rig Veda, the Atharvaveda lifted *kama* to a 'divine' status. In his book *Kama and the Riddle of Desire*,[6] Gurcharan Das shares how *kama* is the subject of many great texts, from the Vedas and Brahmanas to the pioneering *Upanishads*, which sought to further understand the order of the natural world, the self, and the soul. The *Brihadaranyaka Upanishad* says:

> *You are what your deep, driving desire is*
> *As your desire is, so is your will*
> *As your will is, so is your deed*
> *As your deed, so is your destiny*[7]

The epic Mahabharata shares 40 chapters about Kama's nature and the message: 'desire is the essence of life'[8] – where 'the delight that the mind and heart experience in enjoying the objects of the natural world of the five senses is kama.'[9]

The stories of Krishna's love for Radha and the many *gopis* (consorts with unconditional devotion) dances with the idea of *kama*. The Bhagavad Gita concludes that desire itself is not an issue; rather, attachment to the fruits of that desire is what causes suffering.

Through many more centuries of sacred text and mythology, *kama* took on a new meaning, moving from its original cosmic nature to also refer to sensual pleasure enjoyed through the senses and erotic desire.

Das beautifully notes, 'Kama is not only the joy of sensual attraction but also the aesthetic delight one feels while, say, beholding a Mughal miniature of great beauty,' reminding us how *kama* is the joy we feel through art and the senses. He goes on to say that 'instinctual desire travels from our senses to our imagination, whence it creates a fantasy around a specific individual; these fantasies are the source of intense pleasure which happens to be the other meaning of *kama*.'[10]

Through different texts and paths, you'll see *kama* represented in both sexual and sensual, as well as asexual, formats. This divine energy of desire was also given the name *shakti*, which we have discovered as the source of sensuality within us and within the natural world.

Kama also exists in the four *purusharthas*, which translate from Sanskrit as the 'goals' or 'virtues' of human existence, or 'the soul's purpose.' *Kama* held such value in ancient India that desire and enjoyment of the senses was given a role as one of these four goals or pillars of life. It shared this with the other three: *dharma* (righteous duty or virtuous living), *artha* (material wealth), and *moksha* (spiritual liberation). In this philosophy, pleasure and desire are not an afterthought; they are considered a duty in life, and without them, life is neither wholesome nor complete. This isn't a 'duty' to fulfill your partner's or society's needs. This is about you, your soul desire, and its enjoyment, independent of anyone else.

Kama wasn't just about momentary desire; it was built upon the foundation that happy, stable relationships (filled with sensual pleasure) made for a happy, stable society; together, these would bring us to experience *moksha*, ultimate spiritual freedom.

Whitney Wheelock, a teacher I encountered on the nondual Tantric path, would argue, 'Freedom from what?', as he reminds us that *ananda* (bliss, or our true nature) can be experienced in the everyday as divinity manifesting itself. In fact, the Tantric path is one that allows your relationships to become a temple, your work to become a prayer, and your body to be a safe home for divine *leela* (play).

This leads us to Vatsyayana's famous Kama Sutra,[11] another greatly misunderstood export from India that was written in the 3rd century CE. Scholars believe Vatsyayana's intention was to highlight *kama* as one of the four *purusharthas*. He compiled these *sutras* through the understanding that *kama* is not only a cosmic energy, but also a sensual energy that can be cultivated within.

Sensual pleasure and desire also transformed from a divine concept into an art form that deserved study, literature, and guidance. Contrary to our contemporary understanding, the Kama Sutra's groundbreaking attitudes are not predominantly sex positions, though these are the aspects that have been cherry-picked for our general amusement. The text is the oldest and most notable of a group of texts on erotic love known as the Kama Shashtras.

The Kama Sutra is made up of seven books that each describe a different form of pleasure; only one chapter in one of these books refers to sexual positions.

Overall, the Kama Sutra forms a guide to the art of living well, and the true nature of achieving love and enjoyment through relationships. It speaks volumes about partnership, desire, and sensuality. Other parts of the text present insight into what society and relationships looked like almost two thousand years ago, during the Gupta empire, as they include navigating relations with concubines and seducing the wives of others.

Though we may have moved on from certain aspects of the text in the 21st century, the essence of this treatise of love and desire remains relevant today.

This would be a good time to introduce you to the playful god and goddess of desire and pleasure, Kamadeva and Rati, who are responsible for sensual or sexual longings.

Kamadeva and Rati: The God and Goddess of Desire

Kamadeva is handsome, wrapped in a red embroidered cloth around his waist and drawn in a carriage pulled by two tropical parrots. His skin is green, and he's bathed in jewels dripping down his body. He's often accompanied by his consort, Rati, who represents sensual pleasure. The Atharvaveda considers both deities to be the wielders of creative power in the universe.

Kamadeva holds a bow made of sugarcane, and his arrows are made of five fragrant flowers: jasmine, the white and blue lotus, and flowers from the Ashoka tree and the mango tree. Each of the five flowers represents one of the five senses; Kamadeva shoots his targets with these flowers to infuse them with love and desire.

In one myth, the gods entrust Kamadeva to wake the ascetic yogi, Shiva, from his deep meditation, because the only way to save the world is if Shiva sires a son. Knowing that a yogi who has given up the world is unlikely to procreate, the gods need Kamadeva to fire his arrows at Shiva.

Kamadeva fires his arrows and awakens Shiva's senses, drawing him from his deep meditation to fall in love with Parvati. Parvati and Shiva make love across the cosmic ages, giving rise to the Tantric practices. One day, Shiva awakens from his slumber and shoots from his third eye a fire that destroys Kamadeva and burns him to ashes. Shiva smothers the ashes over his body, representing his relinquishing of desire.

But with Kamadeva gone, all love, longing, and desire vanish from the world. Parvati is deeply concerned with this, as dispelling desire not only means sensual enjoyment and pleasure are gone, but that the drive to perpetuate humanity is gone, along with the desire for the universe to exist at all.

Parvati and Shiva's relationship is a great teacher. She speaks with him and asks him to bring desire back to the world, as all of life is suffering without it, and will eventually die out. Shiva raises Kamadeva from the ashes. He then returns to his cosmic union with Parvati, and humanity is restored.

The famous Vigyan Bhairav Tantra is composed of 112 meditations offered from Shiva to Parvati, after she witnesses all the sufferings in the world. It is one of the most beautiful texts on sensuality. I particularly love the poetic translation called *The Radiance Sutras*, by Lorin Roche,[12] shared in the epigraph at the beginning of this book.

The Paradox of Desire

It isn't only Victorian prudishness that quashed desire. The paradox of desire rests at the heart of esoteric spiritual debate. After all, desire is something that seems endless; fulfilling one desire automatically generates a new desire.

In India, some spiritual teachers decided desire was a *raga*, or negative mental state creating an obstacle to spiritual growth. They believed it was to be avoided or eliminated entirely.

In another myth, Shiva says he has no need for desire, as he is a great meditator; Parvati becomes so enraged by this, she transforms into the goddess Kali and reminds him in her great power, fury, and rage, that even his meditation is born from desire. So, whether desire is good or bad is not the question. Desire simply *is*, even on the spiritual path. And if it's a part of our human existence, then it's best we understand and befriend it.

Some desires are our friends and lead us to live happy, healthy, fulfilled lives. Other times, our desires lead us to harm ourselves and others. Not all desires support living harmoniously in society, community, and family, but that doesn't mean they don't exist.

Remember, connection to our desires does not necessarily mean carrying them into our actions or trying to rid ourselves of them. It's more about being in conversation with them, feeling their charge, and understanding them.

In doing so, we can be empowered to navigate them and have an empowered choice about whether or not to act on them, rather than letting them act on us.

Things get messy when we deny the existence of desire. According to Freud's wish fulfillment theory,[13] when desires are repressed by guilt and taboo, the ego and superego relegate them to the unconscious, the part that drives our speech, action, and choices under the surface. As we explored earlier in the book, this is known as a *vasana*, which literally means 'wishing or desiring,' and derives from our *samskaras*, or imprints we collect from experiences in this and other lifetimes. Our *vasanas* can drive us into addictions, cravings, aversion, harm to ourselves, and harm to others. This is why Tantra works to help process and remove them, by understanding the root cause of the problem.

Depression is desire pressed down until we forego the will to want or to do anything at all, which leads to disconnection from our senses and soul. The whole world becomes bland and void of sensuousness. Understanding our desires is a helpful tool in feeling more alive, sensual, and able to express them freely within ourselves, with honesty. It's also how we learn to live and love more intimately.

Let's look at some ways to release our voices, connect to desire within, and express them to others.

▼ Activities ▼

Bija Mantras

A *bija mantra* is a sound containing a short, one-word syllable that can be chanted aloud or silently. *Bija* means 'seed.' *Bija mantras* are powerful tools to stimulate specific points in the body and to unblock and open our voices, and expand and direct the flow of *kundalini shakti* through the body by activating specific frequencies that bring the *chakras* into balance along our Sensual Rivermap.

You can center your attention on the area and chant the sound internally (*madhyama*) or open your voice and chant aloud. You can find the *mantras* to chant along with via the SOSA website.

Bija Mantra	Chakra	Pronunciation
Lam	*Mulhadhara* (root)	Lum
Vam	*Svadhistana* (sacral center)	Vum
Ram	*Manipura* (solar plexus)	Rum
Yam	*Anahata* (heart)	Yum
Ham	*Vishuddha* (throat)	Hum
Om	*Ajna* (third eye)	Aum
Silence	*Sahasrara* (crown)	Silence

Humming and Horselipping

This is an incredible way to self-soothe, calm the nervous system, and release any pent-up knots of energy in the mouth, jaw, lips, throat, and ears. Humming is self-explanatory, but toning the hum to different ranges can be a fun way to explore, expand, and strengthen the voice, as well as relax the vagus nerve.

Horselipping is often used in labor, to relax contractions in the pelvic floor, cervix, and perineum. It is done by totally relaxing the lips and blowing a good amount of air through them with some pressure; this allows the lips to flap together, like the lips of a horse. It's like blowing raspberries and can be done while visualizing the pelvic floor softening.

Activity: Bee Breath

Brahmari pranayama, or bee breath, is the energetic practice of humming to relax the nervous system and thoughts through the power of sound vibration.

1. Close your eyes and press your thumb on the cartilage of your ears to close them; the rest of your fingers can wrap and rest over your eyes to form a blindfold.

2. Tuning out these senses, take a deep breath and start to hum, making the sound of a bee, until you have finished your breath.

3. Begin again and do 5–10 rounds to begin with, increasing as you become more accustomed to the practice.

4. To complete, remove your hands and meditate on the sensations within.

Tip: Try different pitches and listen to the vibration move around the mind and body.

SENSFUL Method with Desire

Your sensations carry the message of desire through your body into their expression or completion, which leads to satisfaction. This starts with self-empathy. When we express and accept our desires, this leads to deeper self-knowledge and sensuality.

Let's look at the steps for communicating desires to ourselves. There is a different tool for expressing desires to another.

1. **S – Safety:** Ground the body by connecting to the senses and setting up in a safe and private space.

2. **E – Evoke:** Attune to what you're feeling right now, emotionally and physically, and journal about it. Try not to judge yourself; just write with no bounds.

3. **N – Notice:** Become aware of any sensations coming up for you as you connect to this.

4. **S – Sublimate:** Say to yourself: *I can feel the heaviness in my legs and tension in my shoulders. What do I need right now?*

5. **F – Free:** Journal about what you need and desire: *I see the heaviness in my legs and tension in my shoulders right now. I would really like a massage and to adapt how long I sit at my desk at work.*

6. **U – Understand:** Accept this answer with nonjudgment and empathy. Think about whether the acceptance and expression felt like they were enough, and whether acting on the desire will lead you closer to your soul or further away from it. You may also choose to plan how to fulfill your desire. Or, you may feel comfortable having recognized and expressed it within yourself, without carrying it out.

7. **L – Love:** Bring the nervous system back into harmony by balancing your breath, grounding, dancing, or reciting affirmations: *My desires are valid. I am worthy of my desires. My desires are my soul speaking through me.*

Expressing Desire to Others

Expressing your desires may require the participation or acceptance of another, or negotiation. There are two incredible methods for expressing our desires and needs that engage the participation of another while remaining true to who we are through the art of conversation. Having these conversations with a framework that safely holds both people, with active listening and mirroring, can lead to deep feelings of satisfaction.

It is helpful for both people to have a copy of the framework and an intention for the conversation, as well as time boundaries around it.

The activities can be completed alone or with a partner, friend, colleague, or family member.

Remember, whether or not your desire moves into fruition, its expression can be deeply connecting and freeing. Both modalities have entire books of their own, which I invite you to explore.

Nonviolent Communication (NVC), by Marshall Rosenberg[14]

Use the following framework for your conversation:

1. **Observations:** *When I...* (referring to a factual situation between you both, not a reason to blame the other)

2. **Feelings:** *I feel...* (emotion or sensation rather than thought/judgment/perception)

3. **Needs:** *What I need is...* (refer to list of universal human needs on NVC website)

4. **Requests:** *Would you be willing to...* (make a suggestion for a response – see SMART requests in Step 5)

5. **Mirroring:** The person repeats back what you say, word for word, which leads to the sensation of your needs and desires being heard and connects the listener to empathy. The request can lead to acceptance, negotiation, or simply understanding. The key is speaking in 'I' rather than 'you' statements, which removes blame and 'violence,' and leads to empowering, vulnerable conversations.

   Example 1: *When I was at the restaurant last night and saw you on your phone, I experienced loneliness, because it reminded me of when my parents were too busy to sit at dinner with me when I was a child. I have a need for connection. Would you be willing to have phone-free time while we're eating dinner at the restaurant next week?*

Example 2: *When I was in bed with you last night at 10 p.m. and the TV was on until 12 a.m., I felt angry and upset, because I have a need for rest before my meetings in the morning. Would you be willing to watch TV in the living room on weekdays after 10 p.m.?*

Imago Dialogue SMART Method, by Dr. Harville Hendrix and Dr. Helen LaKelly Hunt[15]

This tool is from Imago Therapy, which is based on transforming conflict into opportunity for healing and growth. Hendrix and Hunt are couples therapists, but this method can be used to express desire in any form of relationship. The conversation is based on agreeing to talk in a specific time frame; listening and reflecting back (mirroring); summarizing to make sure you've heard all as intended; validating the thought, desire, or expression as the other's truth; and empathizing to deepen the connection.

While all these steps are for deeper connection, this isn't necessarily about agreeing with the other person. The framework for expressing and requesting our desires, needs, and boundaries can utilize the SMART framework below. This can be helpful in the 'would you be willing to' section (Step 4) of the previous exercise.

1. **S - Specific:** Be specific about what you need, not general. Instead of saying, 'I need more touch,' specify where, for how long, and with detail, so the other person knows what you need and desire, and knows how to execute it, if they agree to. For example, 'I'd like you to stroke my hair softly before we fall asleep.'

2. **M - Measurable:** This can refer to frequency. For example, 'On Mondays...'

3. **A - Achievable:** In order for it to be achievable, chunk it down into a reasonable amount of time. For example, 'During the first 10 minutes of watching this program, or during dinnertime at weekends...'

4. **R – Relevant:** Is the request relevant to the frustration or need (frustration might focus on lack of touch, whereas need will focus on the desire for intimacy)?

5. **T – Timely:** Specify an exact time frame in which to fulfill the request. For example, 'Would you be willing to try that for the next two weeks?'

Integration

1. How do you feel expressing your opinions, truth, desires, and thoughts?

2. What did you learn about *kama* (desire) in your own upbringing?

3. What did you learn from the myth of Kamadeva, Shiva, and Parvati? Do you relate to any of the characters or their situations?

4. Try a conscious communication technique or practice by journaling about it first.

Key Takeaways

~ To desire is to be alive. When desire ceases, life ceases.

~ Desires that are repressed remain active within us, seeking expression or gratification, even if they're denied. That's why it's best to develop a relationship with our desires, so we can either consciously choose to act on them or channel them through other expressions.

~ The expression of desire, when it is both spoken and heard, leads to wholeness, satisfaction, and completion in our lives. Its home is in our communication center, *Vishuddha chakra*.

~ The anatomical structure of the voice box and the *yoni* (Sanskrit for 'vulva, womb, cervix, and vagina') are incredibly similar. Over the course of our lives, each time our voice and desire are shut down, the message is stored and mirrored in both the pelvis and throat.

~ *Kama*, or desire, is the subject of many sacred texts, ranging from *kama* as a cosmic force to an expression of sensual pleasure.

~ The ancient text known as the Kama Sutra is a guide to the art of living well, and the true nature of achieving love and enjoyment through our relationships.

~ The god of desire and pleasure, Kamadeva, is responsible for sensual or sexual longings, and appears in important myths about the dance between Shiva (consciousness) and Shakti (power), who both join together to create life.

CHAPTER 12

Meeting the Lover Within

There's a place somewhere between effort and surrender. In that place, *shiva* meets *shakti*, and consciousness meets power. It is in this meeting that the small struggles of separation dissolve, love emerges, and we finally remember *sat chit ananda*: that our true nature is bliss.

Tantra reveals to us that we need not look elsewhere to find love. We need not wait for a partner to activate our sensuality. It reminds us of the pleasure that springs from connecting with the divine within. This path draws together all parts of our inner world that have split and cascaded into opposite directions, including the parts we both love and hate about ourselves. Understanding universal polarities is the basis of this practice; the polarities merge until they're experienced as a tool for our spiritual evolution.

Harmony and union of the lover within invites us to reflect that union out into the world and attract people, places, and opportunities that honor this connection. The positive charge of sensual energy creates space for deeper pleasure, vitality, and intimacy within ourselves and within our relationships. In this final chapter, you'll meet the lover within and learn to cultivate and channel your sensual energy to flow into your sex, love, and relationships.

Unraveling into Openness

For many years, I hopped from one relationship to another, leaving before I had to unravel myself – scared that if I truly were to, I might be rejected. The truth was, I hadn't unraveled those parts within myself and given myself the love, affirmation and acceptance I was seeking.

Tantra came into my life and offered me a way to open my heart, so I could experience myself as whole. This occurred through Tantric practices and philosophy, as well as working with the deities. It inspired a love deeper than I knew was possible. First, my relationship with myself changed, and then, so did my relationships with others.

As my love for wholeness, rawness, and realness grew deeper, my connections with others grew more whole, more raw, and more real. After a break from dating, I attracted a man, whom many of you know goes by the name Mr. X, into my life. He possessed the deepest consciousness in which I could experience my power. And of course, appreciating the polarity in our differences rather than seeking someone 'exactly' like me, who 'got' me without explanation, gave rise to a deeply Tantric experience that influenced just about every aspect of our intimate relationship, including sex!

The *Yoni*

As you discovered in the last chapter, *yoni* is a Sanskrit word that means 'source or origin' and also refers to the entirety of the female sex organs, including the womb, vagina, and vulva. It's the visual representation of *shakti* and the descending creative force of the inner and outer cosmos. It's often depicted as a downward-pointed triangle.

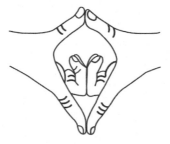

Yoni mudra

You'll see the figure appear throughout different cultures in both natural and human-made forms, from Stonehenge in England, to the Utroba Caves in Bulgaria, to sculptures worshipped across India.

The *yoni* is not used as a derogatory word, such as *pussy* or *cunt*, but as a visual and vocal representation of the dynamic creative power, *shakti*, with sacred value.

In his book *The Yoni*, Rufus C. Camphausen offers the context of the word from Sanskrit, where each letter holds a particular meaning, as well as philosophical value and symbolism. The alphabet of Sanskrit is known as Devanagari, which itself means 'language of the gods.' The word created by the four letters *y*, *o*, *n*, and *i* represent the following:[1]

▼ *y* = the animating principle, the heart, the true self, and union

▼ *o* = preservation, brightness

▼ *n* = love, desire, consciousness, to shine, to pervade, pain and sorrow

▼ *i* = lotus, motherhood, menstrual cycle, nakedness, emptiness, pearl

In Chapter 3, we encountered the menstruating *yoni* that rests in the temple of Kamakhya and is revered by thousands of devotees each year. In the same way, the *yoni* of each individual is its own sacred *shakti pitha*, or altar of creative, sexual, and sensual power.

The symbol of the *yoni* is often worshipped with a pooja. The *yoni pooja* can be done with a sculpture, painting, *yantra* (sacred geometric diagram), or with the *yoni* itself. The *pooja* varies across different traditions. One of them honors the *yoni* with the five elements by pouring five liquids over it: yogurt to represent earth, honey to represent fire, milk to represent air, oil to represent ether, and water to represent itself. The liquids are purified by the *yoni* and then offered as a *prasad* (a consecrated offering from the deity) back to those who offer it. As the symbol of creative power, it is often a site of co-created manifesting potential for its devotees. We don't need a physical womb in order to honor this creative potential.

In the Sensual Rivermap, it's usually placed in *Svadhistana*, the sacral *chakra*, which is connected to the water functions in the body – as the womb also holds fluids of menstrual blood, cervical mucus, sexual waters, and the amniotic waters of childbirth. But the *yoni* is also the entry point of *prana* into the body; it touches the earth element, so it's inextricably intertwined with *Mulhadhara*, the root *chakra*.

This overlapping bridge is surveyed in books such as *Yoni Shakti* by Uma Dinsmore-Tuli and *Laya Yoga* by Shyam Sundar Goswami. This unique meeting point of earth and water in the *yoni* is known as *yonisthana chakra*, meaning 'the place of the *yoni*.'[2] The practices for its healing, nourishment, awakening, and expansion are found both within it and also in the sacred connection between the feet and the earth, as well as through the river that connects the *yoni* with the spiritual heart, via the *yoni-hrydaya-nadi*. All of these can be accessed through Tantra Yoga, *mantra*, *pranayama*, *bhakti*, and grounding — and in fostering a deeper connection between the heart, feet, voice, and *yoni*.

In Taoism, the empresses and emperors of the Far East have long cultivated sexual and sensual energy in a similar way to Tantra. Where the Tantric and yogic paths call this *kundalini shakti*, the Taoist path calls it *ching*, the sexual essence that can be transformed and transmuted into *qi* (life force or energy) to bring us deeper states of harmony, health, and wholeness.

Taoism presents the three gateways of the *yoni*, which are sites where we can release what is not emotionally, energetically, and physically needed each month, through the liquids and elixirs of this area. These gateways also form a doorway inward, in which we share our inner cosmos with another. As such, the gateways bring awareness to everything that comes in contact with the *yoni*, from menstrual products to thoughts, to people and the energy we share with them in this sacred space. It's a gift to be invited into the *yoni* to experience its magnificent creative power.

Giving names to the different parts of our *yoni* is one of the first steps in reclaiming its power. If you were trying to get the attention of a friend on the other side of the room, wouldn't you call their name? When we know the names of the different parts of our *yoni*, we begin to sense the areas more deeply and they respond with their sensation and sacred messages.

If you haven't familiarized yourself with the pleasure anatomy of the *yoni*, here we'll explore both the physical and Taoist gateways to accessing reservoirs of *kundalini shakti*. Getting to know our gateways can help to inform how we are feeling, and which gate we'd like to invite ourselves or anyone else into, if at all. The gateways can hold incredible pleasure, but also pain and numbness that can be encountered along the way.

A simple question when passing through each gateway is: *Does this gateway feel ready to receive?* Then, wait for a response. This makes for sensual connection with our bodies, deeper trust, and even deeper intimacy.

The Three Gateways

When entering the gateways of the *yoni*, the process should begin with relaxation of the nervous system through grounding (*Mulhadhara*). This can occur through massage of the whole body; scanning and relaxing from the top of the head to the toes; engaging in conversation to discuss how you are feeling and being mirrored back; and focusing on the breath, observing the senses, and becoming present.

1. The first gateway is the clitoris, which is believed to have at least 10,280 nerve endings,[3] over double the amount in the penis. The sole purpose of the clitoris in the human body is pleasure. Only the very tip of the clitoris, the glans, is actually visible, in the clitoral hood. Inside the body, the clitoris also extends into the shape of an upside-down V that has two vestibular bulbs and crura (hind) legs behind the skin that straddle the urethral tube, which you pee from, and the vagina. When the clitoris is aroused, the bulbs engorge and can even double in size. *Yonis* get erections, too! The bulbs contract around the urethral tube and stop any bacteria from getting up into the urethra and causing urinary tract infections. The urethral tube is closed, opening the gateway to the vulva and vaginal entrance, which is lubricated by the Bartholin's glands, two tiny holes at either side of the vaginal opening. Many recurring infections could

be prevented if the *yoni* were fully prepared, lubricated, and aroused before penetration. For the bulbs to fill fully, it takes around 45 minutes.

2. The second gateway is only to be approached once the first gate is open — meaning the tissues are engorged; there is enough lubrication; and the heart, body, and mind feel ready for penetration by a finger, toy, crystal wand, or penis. The second gate is located two to three inches inside the upper wall, close to the belly button. It has a lumpy texture and is sometimes known as the G-spot, but is a tube of sensation rather than one specific spot. Tapping the area can evoke a lot of *kundalini shakti* within the body, which can be drawn up using breath for our healing and expansion. This gateway has its own waters; when the fluids are released, this is known as 'squirting.' Mal Weeraratne's book *Emotional Detox Bodywork: A Woman's Guide to Healing and Awakening* calls this *yoni crying*, a birthright for each person with a *yoni*, releasing stored emotion and trauma from the entire body.[4]

3. The third gateway is the cervix, which is directly connected to the vagus nerve and can hold deep pleasure, but also deep pain, trauma, and even numbness. The cervix moves through the menstrual cycle — during ovulation, it is higher up, and during menstruation, it is lower down, which is why the sensual tracking we explored in Chapter 4 can be helpful. As the space, texture, and wetness within the *yoni* changes through the month, we can feel into whether penetration would be welcome during certain times or not. The cervix also has its own waters; when it's released, it's less 'squirting' and more 'flushing' or 'gushing,' like opening the dams of a river. This gateway connects to the heart and forms a direct path to

release trauma and emotions stored in the body. There are two spots on either side of the cervix, known as the A-spot.

When we're in touch with our bodies, sensations, and senses, we know what we have and how we feel; moreover, we can ask for what we want and express what we don't want. This is empowered sensual wisdom as a pathway to unlocking a vital sensual energy that can be used for our nourishment, healing, creativity, manifestation, and spiritual journey.

The Lingam

Lingam (also called *linga*) translates from Sanskrit as 'chief mark' or 'characteristic,' although it is commonly used to refer to the *Shiva lingam*, which is a form in worship of the god Shiva. The *Shiva lingam* is often seen in temples as an upright, conical phallic shape; however, *lingams* can come in different shapes and sizes, including triangular or columnar. To devotees, a *Shiva lingam* represents the cosmic principle of generative, ascending energy.

There are 12 famous *Shiva lingams* in special temples in India, known as *Jyotirlingams*. In his book *Inner Tantric Yoga*, David Frawley reminds us that in yoga philosophy, the term 'linga refers to the subtle body which is the dominant principle in our nature over the physical body. The linga is chiefly a place where energy is held, generated and sustained.'[5]

We have a *prana lingam*, the force that holds up the physical body. We have the *buddhi lingam*, through which our intelligence provides insight and intuition. We have the *atma lingam*, the force that keeps our higher self in a state of transcendence. Basically, a *lingam* refers to anything that upholds. The spine, for example, carries the upward flow of *shiva* energy and the downward spiral of *shakti* energy. In popular culture, the *lingam* is also another word for the penis and sex organs.

The upholding principle is also found in the penetrating generative force of plants and animals, including humans. It is the energy that pollinates, which is why the *lingam* is often associated with the penis. In the left-hand path of Tantra, sex as a meditative tool for evolution was only offered to a serious *sanyasin* who had mastered their energy, under the guidance of a teacher, to understand and transmute it and channel *shiva* and *shakti* to find union.

For this reason, many temples will present a sculpture representing the union of the *yoni* and the *lingam* to symbolize the two forces of the universe. Sometimes, the union is represented in figurative paintings, with an image of two seated figures in an interlocking embrace with their arms and legs around each other; this posture is known as *yabyam*. The union is also seen through the Sri Yantra, which reflects the pulsing geometric principle of the universe.

In Taoism, a sister path of Tantra, teachers such as Mantak Chia have drawn the ancient knowledge of how to cultivate the power held in the physical *lingam* for sexual energy to nourish the mind, body, and organs. For *lingams*, the sperm is the storehouse of *ching* energy and is stored in the testicles.

In his book *Taoist Secrets of Love*, Mantak Chia shares how a single ejaculation has 200 to 500 million sperm cells, all with the potential to become a human being. A single ejaculation is enough to populate the entire United States if each sperm were to fertilize an egg.[6] The energy in this, as you can imagine, is a great resource; if we don't plan on creating a child each time we have sex, this energy can be drawn inward.

The Taoist path teaches that conservation of sexual energy is essential for both solo and dual cultivation. This is why energy depletes and feelings of union dissipate after ejaculation. Orgasm and ejaculation are, in fact, two separate processes. Orgasm is an energetic process whereby energy can be transmuted through the body. Ejaculation is the process of physically releasing sperm.

This doesn't mean that one should never ejaculate; it means doing it consciously, at specific intervals. A rough calculation can be done according to your age, divided by five, resulting in the number of days between ejaculations. The younger you are, the more quickly energy can be regenerated; the older you are, the more energy is required to move inward to nourish and heal (and even to lengthen one's life span), so less frequent ejaculation is recommended. If you're 40, for example, it's recommended that you ejaculate every eight days; after the age of 60, ejaculation is not recommended, as *ching* should be conserved for vitality; however, orgasm is fine. Taoism teaches us that orgasm need not happen simultaneously with ejaculation.

Mal Weeraratne's *Emotional Detox Bodywork: A Woman's Guide to Healing and Awakening* estimates that 80 percent of trauma in the body is stored in the prostate.[7] Upon ejaculation, sperm travels from the testicles through tubes that pass through the prostate; this massages the prostate and creates sensations associated with the release of stress and tension.

The prostate can be blocked with emotion and trauma. The classic phrase 'boys don't cry' means the pea-size prostate can hold a lifetime of emotions that have never been expressed. Excessive masturbation, anger, or sexual appetite may be a response to the body's natural need to offload the trauma energy held in the prostate. But the prostate can be released without ejaculation, through a process of deep bodywork. The body needs to be relaxed, calm, and grounded through physical touch, massage, breath, or conversation.

Relaxation of the body to ground through the root is similar to the first step of relaxing the *yoni*. Massage is firmer and deeper, to soften the body and calm testosterone. The heart, mind, and body need to be open and willing. The prostate can be accessed by a bodyworker through massaging the perineum, which is the skin between the penis and the anus, or directly through the sphincter. As there is so much prejudice around this, it becomes a practice and area that gets repressed. Tantra gives us ways to look beyond 'normal' and embrace all aspects of the body as equal in sacred nature.

Now, let's meet another divine figure that helps us move beyond labels.

Ardhanarishvara/Ardhanari

Ardhanarishvara translates to 'the lord who is half woman' and is a form of Shiva combined with his consort, Parvati, to become Ardhanari. The right side represents Shiva, the masculine, consciousness, and stillness. This side is accompanied by his cow, Nandini. The left side represents Shakti, the feminine, power, and flow. This side is accompanied by her tiger, Somnandi.

The right side has hair of matted locks, tiger skin covering his loins, and serpents as ornaments. The left side has neatly combed and knotted hair, eyes outlined in black kohl, a silk *sari* draped around her body, jewelry, and a red foot dyed with henna. Together, the sides are joined at the center line of their bodies by the third eye and *atilak* (red dot) adorning the middle of the forehead.

Ardhanarishvara represents the union of polarities, Shiva and Shakti, consciousness and power, masculine and feminine energies that live within each human body, no matter the gender. The *Brihadaranyaka*

Upanishad says that *purusha* (spirit) splits into two parts, and the two parts make love to produce all life in the universe.

Another myth from the Shiva Purana shares how the creator god, Brahma, first created male beings and then asked them to create others, but they failed to do so. Shiva appeared in front of him in androgynous form and helped Brahma to realize his omission — female beings were necessary for life on Earth, and the two energies of the universe are inseparable.

This divine being represents wholeness beyond duality, beyond man and woman. It symbolizes the unity of opposites in the universe, a theory more recently explored by the field of quantum science. *Purusha* is the *shiva* principle of consciousness, and *prakriti* is *shakti* and the active force of matter; both are in a continual dance with each other as waves and vibrations that, when together, create the illusion that we are solid forms.

Today in India, Ardhanarishvara is the patron of the third gender known as *hijra*. *Hijras* are the trans community who have been a part of the diverse civilization of India for as long as it has existed. They represent the union of *shiva* and *shakti* polarities within, and the freedom of sexuality and gender. *Hijras* played a significant role in ancient texts, including the Mahabharata, the Ramayana, and the Kama Sutra.

Hijras are still a part of the Indian community today, revered and celebrated but also victims of hate crimes and discrimination. British rule sought to criminalize the *hijra* community, along with many of the other views that did not align with the Victorian era. These laws were repealed after India gained independence, but the discrimination and uneasiness remain. As we move to reconnect with practices of pleasure and love, this is a reminder of the freedom ancient civilizations offered in the expression of gender and sexuality. When we move away from labels of how 'men' and 'women' should experience pleasure, we find liberation and playfulness, as we cultivate deeper love and sensuality.

Modern Attachment

Attachment theory was introduced by psychoanalyst John Bowlby[8] and expanded by Mary Ainsworth. It shares that we're born with a need to form bonds with our primary caregiver. The availability and quality of this caregiving forms the basis of our emotional bonds and relationships in life as adults.

Secure attachment means that, in early childhood, we have dependable caregivers, which creates a secure base for us to explore the world and to feel comfortable depending on ourselves and others. Insecure attachment in childhood will lead to difficulty engaging in intimacy and forming healthy relationships in adulthood. This might take the form of:

1. **Avoidant attachment:** avoiding emotional relating, commitments, and intimacy

2. **Anxious attachment:** being needy/clingy, or having difficulty being alone

3. **Disorganized attachment:** having a fearfully avoidant nature and extreme difficulty trusting others

The premise is that we unconsciously find in our partners all of our unmet needs from childhood, repeating what has happened to us because it feels familiar. Someone who's avoidant will often find someone who's anxious to repeat the cycle with. This is why 'love at first sight' can often feel like a spark gets ignited with someone you've known your entire life. This person usually has the qualities of a caregiver, which is why they feel like home. While this attraction is an unconscious process, understanding your attachment style may help you recognize the polarities within, as well as the polarities you choose in a partner.

Although we can't choose who we grew up with and the attachment style we developed, we can feel empowered in our awareness, which helps us heal our pain and reach for deeper intimacy. In this way, our relationships can become vehicles for healing and evolution.

For example, let's say one partner (Partner A) is anxious and worries their partner will leave them if they haven't responded to a text. The other partner (Partner B) is avoidant and doesn't think twice about getting through a day without texting. If both of them can communicate with each other during the day, this will help to soothe Partner A and heal Partner B's avoidant tendency. At the same time, they can both operate with the understanding that just because Partner B doesn't always respond, doesn't mean the relationship will end – which will help to soothe Partner B and heal Partner A's anxious tendency.

Let's take a deeper look at how this works in ancient love dynamics that include polarities.

Ancient Love Dynamics

The first two *chakras*, *Mulhadhara* and *Svadhistana*, which rule our sexuality and sensuality, imply the existence of polarity. For polarity to exist, there need to be two of something.

Polarity is expansion and contraction, up and down, mind and body, like and dislike, love and hate, left and right, *purusha* and *prakriti*, consciousness and power, self and another. It's a lot like a magnet: When facing one direction, the polarities can pull together; when facing away from each other, they separate. Likewise, polarities are explored in expanding sensual energy and finding inner union with ourselves, our relationships, and the world around us.

If we nourish and charge the polarities within, a
magnetic flow of energy begins to circulate in our
mind, body, and spirit, which can lead us from feelings
of separation to connection with ourselves, each
other, and the divine. This can be felt as pleasure,
love, harmony, connection, and attraction.

When we align with the lover within, we attract the same qualities in a new or existing partner, which supports each other's polarities rather than recycling unhealthy attachment patterns. We attract from a state of wholeness. In relationships, this does not depend on being the same, thinking the same, and doing the same, as is often thought of when 'becoming one' — but rather, celebrating the uniqueness and differences in who you are as individuals together.

Attraction fades when everything in the relationship becomes the same. Attraction heightens when there are differences that are explored, loved, and accepted by the other. The theory of polarities catalyzes the spark of *shakti* and lends itself to a magnificent dance of opposites. As the old adage goes, 'opposites attract,' meaning that lovemaking and relating create a deeply intimate experience.

We can oscillate between our *shiva* and *shakti* energy throughout our lives. For example, when we're children, we may be more in *shakti* mode, or if we have become a provider, we may be required to be in *shiva* mode. The inner lover is felt when we can both give and receive. We are both child and parent — this involves knowing and meeting our needs. The path of Tantra often has connotations of returning to our childlike nature; this doesn't mean being childish, but connecting with the realms of *shakti* that are more receptive, emotional, loving, playful, and intuitive, looked after by the inner guardian who loves and accepts us unconditionally.

In relationships, if you're more in your *shakti* nature, you may find a partner who is more in their *shiva* nature; then, in your relationship, you'll experience a circuit of union through polarity. For example, if one partner is very grounding and one partner is very emotional, the emotions will find a space to ground and the grounded person will be inspired to express their emotions.

If you both play a *shiva* role in your relationship and display grounding, structure, power, and independence, as is often required in a patriarchal society, you may want to play with one person stepping more into their *shakti* by working with the qualities of receiving, softening, surrendering, and flowing, to catalyze attraction. All genders can play with the art of polarities.

Each of the *chakras* is connected primarily to either a *shiva* or *shakti* energy.

▼ **Mulhadhara:** *shiva* energy (grounding, calm, rootedness, safety, stillness)

▼ **Svadhistana:** *shakti* energy (sensuality, emotion, flow, creativity)

▼ **Manipura:** *shiva* energy (power, confidence, self-worth, independence)

▼ **Anahata:** *shakti* energy (love, forgiveness, openness, nonjudgment)

▼ **Vishuddha:** *shiva* energy (expression of truth, listening to truth)

▼ **Ajna:** *shakti* energy (intuition, foresight, imagination)

▼ **Sahasrara:** union (connection with higher power, togetherness, community)

In dual cultivation of *kundalini shakti* with a partner, a couple will use practices to evoke sexual energy in the body; they will then circulate the subtle *kundalini shakti* energy between them and transform it into *prana* to nourish the body and relationship, which create a deeper balance between the *shiva* and *shakti* polarities.

Dual cultivation does not need to include any form of penetration. It is the art of dancing with each other's *shakti* to bring about union within oneself and one's relationship. This can be shared through the art of conversation, breath, and energy, as well as sex.

To deny that sex has a part in Tantra would not be true — it's an inevitable process that's a natural part of living; that's why it's embraced. As you deepen in your sensuality, you will deepen in your sexuality and capacity for love and pleasure, which are part of your sensual wisdom and spiritual evolution.

▼ Activities ▼

SENSFUL Yoni/Lingam Gazing

To become more familiar with the sacredness of your *yoni* or *lingam*, you can practice *yoni/lingam* gazing by yourself or with a partner.

▼ **S – Safety:** Create a private, sacred space and take a few breaths to relax into it and connect to your heart and senses. Take an oil and massage your body from head to toe, inviting all of you to become present and grounded.

▼ **E – Evoke:** Open your legs and take a hand mirror to face your *yoni/lingam*. Can you identify the different parts and their names? How does it look, smell, sound, taste, feel?

▼ **N – Notice:** Be aware of the sensations in your body. What thoughts come up? Allow them to be there but try not to get caught in them; bring yourself back to what you see.

▼ **S – Sublimate:** Breathe any discomfort/pleasure/sensation into the heart and exhale.

▼ **F – Free:** Allow yourself to express what you saw by journaling or speaking aloud.

▼ **U – Understand:** Empathize with where these thoughts/sensations/feelings/memories might have come from.

▼ **L – Love:** Allow yourself to meditate here. Offer yourself positive affirmations, such as: *I am divine consciousness. I am love. I am sacred.* Do this time and again to diffuse judgment, shame, and fear, so you can move into love, acceptance, and pleasure.

Yoni Eggs

Yoni eggs have long been used in Taoist practice among ancient empresses to awaken *ching* and cultivate deeper sensation and strength. *Yoni* eggs can be made from different stones for different qualities and inserted into the *yoni* as a ritual. This can be helpful for learning when the *yoni* is ready, and asserting boundaries before inserting anything into this sacred space.

The stone can be worn in the *yoni* and felt as you move around to evoke and awaken sensation. *Yoni*-egg exercises can also be completed by activating and releasing the pelvic-floor muscles or in accompaniment with a yoga practice. See the SOSA website (*see p.xxi*) for a guide.

Microcosmic Orbit

This was introduced to me through Mantak Chia's School of Universal Healing Tao to provide a circuit for *ching* to flow around the body; clear blocks that manifest from stress, trauma, and diet; and facilitate the use of *ching* for healing, nourishment, and expansion.

1. Stand or sit with your feet flat on the ground and spine straight.

2. Bring your attention to your perineum. As you inhale, gently squeeze or pump to activate the *ching*; using your in-breath, draw the energy up through your spine, through your neck, over the top of your head, and down over your face to the roof of your mouth.

3. Place the tip of your tongue to the roof of your mouth to connect the front and back channels. As you exhale, let the energy wash down the front body, down through your heart, genitals, and back to your perineum.

4. Repeat, creating a circular, healing, nourishing flow of energy orbiting around the body. You can give the orbit a color, sound, smell, taste, or texture.

Edging and Spreading

Casting your attention back to the three gateways, edging and spreading is a practice that can be used to heal numbness, ascertain boundaries, and expand sensation. We explored edging in Chapter 8. Remember, if 10 is an orgasm and 0 is completely neutral, the idea is to bring ourselves to a 7 or 8, so that we can take the *kundalini shakti* and transmute it up the body.

Here, we add the practice of spreading for awakening sensation. You can combine this practice with the microcosmic orbit, and you can do it alone or with a partner.

1. Create a sacred space and relax the body by touching it sensually from head to toe.

2. Start to stimulate the clitoris (pause when you reach a 7 and breathe up and down the body).

3. When and if you feel ready, bring your finger or a crystal wand to the vagina, and ask if you would like to be entered. Wait for a response from your body and listen to the sensations.

4. If the answer is yes, proceed to the second gateway, which is two to three inches within the vagina on the upper wall. It can be stroked with one finger or walked across using two fingers. If there is numbness, return to the clitoris; bring yourself to 6–7, then return to the space where there is numbness. This is the idea of spreading sensation and pleasure.

5. Ask again if you're ready to go deeper toward the cervix. If you're using your fingers, it can help to prop the pelvis up on pillows or even turn over onto your knees. The A-spot is located on either side of the cervix by splitting the fingers in two. If there's numbness, return to somewhere you feel pleasure and sensation, then return to this area when ready.

6. Whenever you approach 7 or 8, pause and breathe up the body through the *chakras*, or use the microcosmic orbit. You can focus on particular areas of the body, mind, or spirit where you would like to transmute the *kundalini shakti* into *prana* to heal, nourish, and expand.

Tantric Date Night

You can journey through the senses and explore the touch of love or the breath of ecstasy together. You can play with polarities through roleplay, as one partner practices giving and the other receiving, before switching; this helps balance *shiva* and *shakti* energy within you and within the partnership, providing deeper sensual connection.

Ideas for date nights are offered in a guided format on the SOSA website. For each date night, create a sacred space through all the elements. Connect with each other through gratitude. Blindfold one partner, and then begin.

1. Journey to the Senses: Use the steps as explored in Chapter 8 for giving and receiving through the senses (see pp.182–183).

2. Touch of Love: Explore different types of touch according to the elements (earth: grounding touch; air: light, whispery touch; fire: fast, hot touch; water: flowing, oily touch; space: the touch of sound vibration).

3. Breath of Ecstasy: Experience full-body orgasm by guiding the breath through the Sensual Rivermap, as explored in Chapter 4.

Meditate on Union: Yabyam

Yabyam is the divine symbol of union between Shiva and Shakti, and it's frequently seen in Tantric deity art. The posture can be assumed as an *asana*, or seat of meditation, for deeper connection.

The larger partner can sit on the ground with legs crossed or outstretched. If this is uncomfortable, use cushions or pillows to support the hips and knees. The other partner will sit on top of the partner with legs wrapped around their waist. The genitals meet at the center (this can be done with clothes on or off), and the arms around the other person's shoulders. If the legs of the bottom partner are open, they can straddle the partner's legs and waist.

Variations on the posture include:

▼ sitting with your foreheads meeting and your eyes closed

▼ sitting with your eyes open, facing each other

▼ breathing in synchronicity with each other

▼ circulating your breath, mouths close together, with one partner inhaling as the other exhales

▼ circulating the energy up and down the *chakras* or by using the microcosmic orbit

▲▲▲

Integration

1. What's your relationship with your *yoni* or *lingam*?

2. What has your relationship to sex, relationships, and pleasure been thus far?

3. What are your positive and negative poles – that is, where do you feel strong/weak, physically/emotionally/energetically, in your Sensual Rivermap?

4. What kinds of partners are you attracted to? Think about past and present partners: What are their positive and negative poles?

5. What sensations arise from the solo/dual love cultivation practices?

KEY TAKEAWAYS

~ Meeting the lover within helps us learn to cultivate and channel sensual energy to flow into our sex, love, and relationships.

~ The *yoni* is the visual representation of *shakti* and the descending creative force of the inner and outer cosmos. It's the sacred symbol of *parashakti* and the universal womb.

~ The three gateways of the *yoni* are sites where we can release emotional, energetic, and physical toxins, through the liquids and elixirs of this area.

~ *Lingam* (also called *linga*) translates from Sanskrit as 'chief mark' or 'characteristic,' although it is commonly used to refer to the penis or the *Shiva lingam*, which is a form in worship of the god Shiva.

~ The Taoist path teaches that conservation of sexual energy, or *ching*, is essential for both solo and dual cultivation.

~ Ardhanarishvara represents the union of polarities, Shiva and Shakti, consciousness and power, masculine and feminine, that live within each human body, no matter the gender.

~ Attachment theory shares that we are born with a need to form bonds with our primary caregiver, but depending on how we were raised, we cultivate 'attachment styles' that determine how we interact with a partner.

~ Exploring polarities within ourselves and with a partner can expand sensual energy and help us find inner union with ourselves and the world around us.

Conclusion

Together, we've whitewater-rafted down the canyons, through the sensuality that innately belongs to us all as a species, in the way we taste, touch, smell, hear, and feel life within and around us. We've run over the rocks that block our access to this sensual life force, and we've discovered new and vast landscapes in which we can use sensual energy for our own expansion.

Whatever you take from here – whether it's a story, a practice, or even just knowing a little more about Tantra and my cultural heritage – my wish and prayer is that it serves to open your heart, your mind, and your body. May you connect more deeply, express more freely, and love more intimately. Because to sense is what makes us human. And it is our human birthright to reclaim our sensuality, so that every dance, every mouthful, every note of music, every step we take, and every touch we give or receive may be a prayer, connecting us to the source of who we are: *shakti*, the dynamic creative power.

Wherever we meet next, whether through words or practice, I thank you for taking this time to expand with me through these pages.

I wish you love, and I wish you well as you continue your sensual journey. Jai Ma!

Acknowledgments

From conception to contractions, I thought my task was to birth a book. But it turns out the book was birthing me. And over the past few years, while I've teethed my way into the process, learned to crawl, wobble, and eventually walk, taking my own tumbles and turns along the way, it is the unconditional support of my village – my partner, family, friends, publisher, agent, and colleagues at the School of Sensual Arts who have created a scaffolding for me to dive head and heart first into bringing these words to life. While I have, quite honestly, become completely lost and found in its process, I have never forgotten the people without whom these pages would be impossible.

I want to thank my beloved, Mr. X, who's spent long drives and late nights listening to my ideas, supporting me with affirmation and kindness, and filling our relationship with infinite hope, adventure, and potential. I love you.

My loving mother, whose unconditional loyalty, care, and courage inspire me. My supportive father, whose journey as an artist, monk, and traveler has influenced my work more than he has ever known.

My brother, for your continued guidance, compassion, and protection without qualm or question; my sister-in-love, for your generosity, conversation, and charisma; Aary and Avani, for sitting on my lap as babies while I built the School of Sensual Arts from our kitchen table.

To my late siblings, Anish and Jalpa, whose young losses have taught me the value of life and led me on this journey in the first place.

My Aunties and Uncles, for paving the way for our family migrating across continents to London — my Masi and Masa, my Mamis and Mamas. My cousins and cousins-in-love, for first and always believing in me. My aunties, uncles, and cousins in India, for kindling in me my love for my roots, with your love, nourishment, and open arms. My Fois and Foas, Kakis and Kakas, bhais and bens.

My late grandparents, Santaben and Chunibhai, who chose to get on the rickety sailboat to Uganda; and to my grandparents in India, Ratilal and Sushila, who carried the creativity, spirit, and practices I continue to share here.

My family-in-love, the Mixes, for the care you've taken in welcoming me, and for your curiosity, interest, and encouraging words in my unusual line of work.

My incredible friends growing up, at university, through courses and across continents — you know who you are. Shoutout to my original Shakti Circle — Ivena, Pagen, Oriana, and Liz — and Jade, from my latest one!

The members and students of the School of Sensual Arts community — your courage and commitment to your practice inspire me and these very pages. My colleagues, Manoj and Rachel, for your support in keeping the school running while I write. Kiran and Gaetano, for birthing its vision in the first place.

My therapist, TH, who has helped me over the years to find language for the experiences I could never find words for.

My teachers, swamiji, and guides, who have shared with me this path, held space for me to experience its practices, and illuminated what was possible.

My incredible agents Sheila Crowley and Rachel Goldblatt at literary agency Curtis Brown, for taking me on with your years of experience and guiding me through this process.

And last but not least, my publisher – Hay House. With your care, belief, and support through the incredible people on your team – Kezia, Julie, Nirmala, and the many others behind the scenes – you've offered me an opportunity that's much more than writing a book: rediscovering page by page, word by word, my voice, which once quivered but now roars.

Endnotes

Epigraph

1. Roche L. The Radiance Sutras: 112 gateways to the yoga of wonder & delight. Boulder, CO: Sounds True; 2014.

Chapter 1: Knowing Your Sensuality

1. Wallis CD. Tantra Illuminated: The Philosophy, History, and Practice of a Timeless Tradition. Mattamayura Press; 2013 pp.125–150.
2. Rubin G. Life in Five Senses. Crown; 2023 pp.11–14.
3. Dinsmore-Tuli U. Yoni shakti: A woman's guide to power and freedom through yoga and tantra. S.L.: Yogawords; 2020 p.266.

Chapter 2: Knowing Your Sensual Power (Tantra)

1. Wallis CD. Tantra Illuminated: The Philosophy, History, and Practice of a Timeless Tradition. Mattamayura Press; 2013 pp.48–50.
2. Imma Ramos, British Museum. Tantra: Enlightenment to revolution. Editorial: London: Thames and Hudson; 2020, pp.18–20.
3. Ibid.

Chapter 3: Knowing Your Sensual Cycle (Ayurveda)

1. Joseph S. Rtu Vidyā. Notion Press; 2020, pp.242–244.
2. Anand S. The arts of seduction. New Delhi: Aleph; 2018, pp.41–50.

Chapter 4: Knowing Your Sensual Rivermap (Yoga)

1. Goswami SS. Layayoga: The definitive guide to the Chakras and Kundalini. Rochester, VT: Inner Traditions; 1999.

2. Walsch ND. Conversations with God, An Uncommon Dialogue: Living in the World with Honesty, Courage, and Love, Volume 1, p.59.

3. Judith A. Eastern Body, Western Mind. Celestial Arts; 2011, pp.35–40.

4. Goswami SS. Layayoga: The definitive guide to the Chakras and Kundalini. Rochester, VT: Inner Traditions; 1999, Chapter 9.

Part II: Your Nurtured Sensuality

1. Goode G. The Direct Path. New Harbinger Publications; 2012, pp.23–27.

Chapter 5: Feeling Shame

1. Zahavi D. Shame. Oxford University Press eBooks [Internet]. 2014 Nov 27 [cited 2023 Oct 12]; 208–40. Available from: https://academic.oup.com/book/6543/chapter/150481926

2. Solan M. The secret to happiness? Here's some advice from the longest-running study on happiness [Internet]. Harvard Health Blog. 2017 [cited 2023 Oct 12]; Available from: https://www.health.harvard.edu/blog/the-secret-to-happiness-heres-some-advice-from-the-longest-running-study-on-happiness-2017100512543

3. Chinnaiyan KM. Shakti Rising. New Harbinger Publications; 2017, p.19.

4. Frawley D. Inner tantric yoga: Working with the universal shakti – secrets of mantras, deities and meditation. Twin Lakes, WI: Lotus; Enfield; 2009, pp.6–8.

5. Jung CG. Instinct and the unconscious. British Journal of Psychology, 1904–1920. 1919 Nov;10(1):15–23.

6. Kempton S. Awakening to Kali. Sounds True; 2014, p.21.

7. Kinsley D. Tantric Visions of the Divine Feminine. University of California Press; 2023, Chapter 1.

8. Dinsmore-Tuli U. Yoni shakti: A woman's guide to power and freedom through yoga and tantra. S.L.: Yogawords; 2020.

9. Kinsley D. Tantric Visions of the Divine Feminine. University of California Press; 2023 p.2–3.

Chapter 6: Feeling Trauma

1. Racism, Mental Health and Trauma Research Round Up [Internet]. UKTC. [cited 2023 Nov 8]; Available from: https://uktraumacouncil. org/research_practice/racism-and-trauma-research

2. McBride PDHL. The wisdom of your body. Finding healing, wholeness, and connection through embodied living. [United States]: Baker Publishing Group; 2021, pp.58–59

3. Chinnaiyan KM. Shakti Rising. New Harbinger Publications; 2017, p.8.

4. van der Kolk B. The body keeps the score: Brain, mind and body in the healing of trauma. New York: Penguin Books; 2014.

5. Levine PA. Waking the tiger: Healing trauma: The innate capacity to transform overwhelming experiences. Berkeley, CA: North Atlantic Books; 1997.

6. Menakem R. My grandmother's hands: racialized trauma and the pathway to mending our hearts and bodies. Las Vegas, NV: Central Recovery Press; 2017, p.5.

7. Porges SW. The polyvagal theory; and The pocket guide to the polyvagal theory. New York: W.W. Norton and Company; 2018.

8. van der Hart O, Dorahy M. Pierre Janet and the Concept of Dissociation. American Journal of Psychiatry. 2006 Sep;163(9):1646.

9. Office for National Statistics. People who were abused as children are more likely to be abused as an adult – Office for National Statistics [Internet]. Ons.gov.uk. 2017. [cited 2023 Nov 8]; Available from: https://tinyurl.com/27bjpxt6

10. Weeraratne M. Emotional Detox Through Bodywork. Authorhouse UK; 2016, pp.28–35.

Chapter 7: Feeling Fear

1. Jeffers S. Feel the Fear... and Do It Anyway. HarperCollins; 2023, pp.188–192.

2. Ibid., pp.13–16.

3. Kempton S. Awakening to Kali. Sounds True; 2014, pp.31–53.

4. American Psychological Association, What is Exposure Therapy? [Internet]. Available from: https://www.apa.org/ptsd-guideline/ patients-and-families/exposure-therapy.pdf

Chapter 8: Feeling Stress

1. Dual Control Model of Sexual Response [Internet]. kinseyinstitute. org. [cited 2023 Nov 8]; Available from: https://kinseyinstitute.org/ research/dual-control-model.php

2. Nagoski E. Come as you are: The surprising new science that will transform your sex life. S.L.: Simon & Schuster; 2021, pp.42–53.

3. Dinsmore-Tuli U, Tuli N. Yoga Nidra Made Easy. Hay House, Inc; 2022, pp.38–40.

4. Lusk J. Yoga Nidra for Complete Relaxation and Stress Relief. New Harbinger Publications; 2015, p.6.

Chapter 9: Meeting the Manifester Within

1. Swart T. The source: The secrets of the universe, the science of the brain. New York, NY: HarperOne; 2019, p.34–38.

2. Judith A. Chakra yoga. Paris: Éditions Médicis; 2015, p.365–366.

3. Staff M. Are Shiva and Shakti the God Equation that Relativists and Quantum Mechanists Seek? [Internet]. Are Shiva and Shakti the God Equation that Relativists and Quantum Mechanists Seek? [cited 2023 Dec 6]. Available from: https://www.myind.net/Home/ viewArticle/are-shiva-and-shakti-the-god-equation-that-relativists-and-quantum-mechanists-seek#google_vignette

4. Langille JJ, Brown RE. The Synaptic Theory of Memory: A Historical Survey and Reconciliation of Recent Opposition. Frontiers in Systems Neuroscience [Internet]. 2018 Oct 26;12. Available from: https://www.ncbi.nlm.nih.gov/pmc/articles/PMC6212519/

5. Anand M. The art of sexual magic. New York: Putnam; 1995.

Chapter 10: Meeting the Creative Within

1. Quaghebeur J, Petros P, Wyndaele JJ, De Wachter S. The innervation of the bladder, the pelvic floor, and emotion: A review. Autonomic Neuroscience. 2021 Nov;235:102868.

2. Rennison N. Freud and Psychoanalysis. Pocket Essentials; 2001.

3. Maslow Abraham H. Emotional blocks to creativity. Journal of Individual Psychology. 1958;14:51–56

4. Sundquist D, Lubart T. Being Intelligent with Emotions to Benefit Creativity: Emotion across the Seven Cs of Creativity. Journal of Intelligence. 2022 Nov 15;10(4):106.

5. Averill JR, Thomas-Knowles C. Emotional creativity. In: Strongman KT, editor. International Review of Studies on Emotion. vol. 1. Wiley; London: 1991. pp. 269–99.

6. Gupta M. Courting Hindustan. Rupa Publications India Pvt Limited; 2023, pp.5–22.

7. Nevile P. Nautch girls of the Raj. Palgrave Pivot; 2009, p.xi.

Chapter 11: Meeting the Desire Within

1. The Larynx, Basic Anatomy — Eastern Virginia Medical School (EVMS), Norfolk, Hampton Roads [Internet]. www.evms.edu. [cited 2023 Oct 17]. Available from: https://www.evms.edu/patient_care/specialties/ent_surgeons/services/laryngology/anatomy/

2. Shoffel-Havakuk H, Carmel-Neiderman NN, Halperin D, Shapira Galitz Y, Levin D, Haimovich Y, et al. Menstrual Cycle, Vocal Performance, and Laryngeal Vascular Appearance: An Observational Study on 17 Subjects. Journal of Voice. 2018 Mar;32(2):226–33.

3. Bos N, Bozeman J, Cate Frazier-Neely. Singing through change: Women's voices in midlife, menopause, and beyond. Suquamish, WA: Studiobos Media; 2020.

4. Ramesowner S. The Vocal-Vaginal Connection [Internet]. Cate Frazier-Neely. 2021 [cited 2023 Oct 17]. Available from: https://www.catefnstudios.com/writings/the-voice-vaginal-connection

5. Agrawala VS, Sayanakarya. Hymn of Creation. 1963, 129th Hymn of the 10th mandala.

6. Das G. Kama. India Allen Lane; 2018, pp.15–20.

7. Śaṅkarācārya, Madhavananda, Upanishads. Brihad-Āranyaka Upanishad. The Brihadaranyaka upanishad,. Mayavati, Almora, Himalyas, Advaita Ashrama; 1950.

8. Rajagopalachari C. Mahabharata. Bombay: Bharatiya Vidya Bhavan; 2002 XII.167.34.

9. Rajagopalachari C. Mahabharata. Bombay: Bharatiya Vidya Bhavan; 2002 IV.33.37.

10. Das G. Kama. India Allen Lane; 2018, pp.10–11.

11. Vatsyayana. The Kama Sutra of Vatsyayana. Kama Shastra Society of London and Benares; 1883.

12. Roche L. The Radiance Sutras: 112 gateways to the yoga of wonder & delight. Boulder, CO: Sounds True; 2014.

13. Freud S. The interpretation of dreams; and On dreams (1900–1901). London: Hogarth Press; 1995.

14. Rosenberg MB. Nonviolent Communication: A Language of Life. 3rd ed. Encinitas, CA: Puddledancer Press; 2015.

15. Hendrix H, LaKelly H. Getting the Love You Want: A Guide for Couples: Third Edition. St. Martin's Griffin; 2019.

Chapter 12: Meeting the Lover Within

1. Camphausen RC. The Yoni. Inner Traditions; 1996.

2. Dinsmore-Tuli U. Yoni shakti: A woman's guide to power and freedom through yoga and tantra. S.L.: Yogawords; 2020, pp.141–142.

3. Uloko M, Isabey EP, Peters BR. How many nerve fibers innervate the human glans clitoris: a histomorphometric evaluation of the dorsal nerve of the clitoris. The Journal of Sexual Medicine. 2023 Jan 30;20(3):247–52.

4. Weeraratne M. Emotional Detox Through Bodywork. Authorhouse UK; 2016.

5. Frawley D. Inner Tantric yoga: Working with the universal shakti – secrets of mantras, deities and meditation. Twin Lakes, Wis.: Lotus; Enfield; 2009.

6. Chia M, Winn M. Taoist Secrets of Love. Aurora Press; 1984.

7. Weeraratne M. Emotional Detox Through Bodywork. Authorhouse UK; 2016.

8. Bowlby J. The Bowlby-Ainsworth attachment theory. Behavioral and Brain Sciences. 1979 Dec;2(04):637–8.

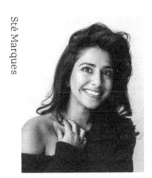

Sté Marques

About the Author

Henika Patel is the founder of the School of Sensual Arts. She's a first-generation British–Indian woman who grew up in a household abundant in the ancient Indian arts. She studied English and French law, but after experiencing depression following a series of losses, she left the corporate world and spent several years studying and learning from incredible guides in India and Asia.

Upon returning to England, Henika began her studies in arts therapy and clinical psychotherapy for individuals and couples, and now combines Tantra and Yoga with Western therapeutic guidelines to create safe spaces for individuals and couples to transform numbness, bust through shame, and find their spark. As an Indigenous practitioner, she's a thought leader and educator on the topic of cultural appropriation of Tantra and Yoga.

Henika also co-founded the charity Sibling Loss Organisation to help people with the unique grief journey of their siblings and cousins. Her work has been featured on Channel 4, Apple TV, and Amazon Prime, by Louis Theroux's production company, and in *Natural Health* and *Women's Health* magazines. Her mission is to create sensory experiences to inspire incredible souls around the world to lean into their desires, embrace their sensuality, and lead life from the heart.

 schoolofsensualarts.co.uk

 henika.x

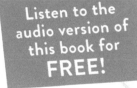

CONNECT WITH
HAY HOUSE
ONLINE

🌐 hayhouse.co.uk   **f** @hayhouse

📷 @hayhouseuk   𝕏 @hayhouseuk

▶ @hayhouseuk   ♪ @hayhouseuk

Find out all about our latest books & card decks • Be the first to know about exclusive discounts • Interact with our authors in live broadcasts • Celebrate the cycle of the seasons with us • Watch free videos from your favourite authors • Connect with like-minded souls

'*The gateways to wisdom and knowledge are always open.*'

Louise Hay